PATIENTS FIRST

How To Save The NHS

Leslie Turnberg

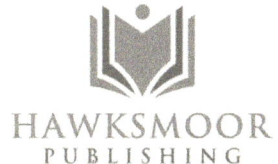

HAWKSMOOR
PUBLISHING

First published in 2024 by Hawksmoor Publishing

Woodside, Oakamoor, ST10 3AE, UK

www.hawksmoorpublishing.com

ISBN: 978-1-914066-47-4

Copyright © Leslie Turnberg 2024

Leslie Turnberg has asserted his right under the Copyright, Designs and Patents Act, 1988, to be identified as the author of this book.

All Rights Reserved. No part of this publication may be reproduced, stored in a retrieval system, or transmitted in any form or by any means, electronic, mechanical, photocopying, recording or otherwise, without the prior permission of the publisher.

A CIP catalogue record for this book is available from the British Library.

This book is sold subject to the condition that it shall not, by way of trade or otherwise, be lent, re-sold, hired out or otherwise circulated without the publisher's prior consent in any form of binding or cover other than that in which it is published and without a similar condition including this condition being imposed on the subsequent purchaser.

Hawksmoor Editorial Review: Dr Charlotte Woodcock

ABOUT THE AUTHOR

Leslie Turnberg was Professor of Medicine and Dean of the Medical School in Manchester before becoming President of the Royal College of Physicians in 1992. He led a review of London's Health Services in 1997, was President of the Medical Protection Society, and was Chair of the Board of the Public Health Laboratory Service before entering the House of Lords in 2000. There, he speaks on health and social care.

Leslie is also the author of a number of other books, including *Forks in the Road*, *Beyond the Balfour Declaration*, *Mandate*, and *An Unreasonable Man*.

ACKNOWLEDGEMENTS

There is not exactly a dearth of books on the health services, but as I watched the failings of my long-admired NHS with some dismay, I felt I could not just stand by. I could not resist the temptation to write about my concerns, and I turned to a number of people whom I respect, half expecting them to urge restraint.

I was surprised and relieved that they did not try to dissuade me, and I am eternally grateful for their encouragement and support. Simon Stevens, who knows something about overseeing a National Health Service, went through the manuscript with an eagle eye and made many vital suggestions. Kay Andrews knows a lot about social care. She chaired a Select Committee on the subject and selflessly gave me of her wisdom. David Dalton, who developed the most successful integrated care system in England, prevented me from making too many errors of judgment and fact. Alexis Ingram gave me a great deal of insight into what it is like to be a GP in the current NHS, while Rebecca Myers selflessly shared her intimate knowledge of working on the front line in local health services and nursing care.

I had enormous support from many friends, but here I mention but two: Jill Pitkeathley and Victor Hoffbrand. Their support has been invaluable.

None of my supporters are responsible for the final product. What is left is, I fear, all my own responsibility.

It is impossible to ignore the invaluable help of my publisher, James Lumsden-Cook, who ensured that I made sense.

Leslie Turnberg, May 2024.

CONTENTS

INTRODUCTION 1

CHAPTER 1: THE ENVY OF THE WORLD? 7
CHAPTER 2: SOCIAL CARE AND CARE
IN THE COMMUNITY 17
CHAPTER 3: PRIMARY CARE 45
CHAPTER 4: CARE IN HOSPITAL 59
CHAPTER 5: MENTAL HEALTH SERVICES 89
CHAPTER 6: MATERNITY SERVICES 97
CHAPTER 7: PUBLIC HEALTH 103
CHAPTER 8: TRUST AND MISTRUST 117
CHAPTER 9: MEDICAL RESEARCH 123
CHAPTER 10: RE-ORGANISATION AND RE-RE-ORGANISATION OF THE NHS 131
CHAPTER 11: FUNDING MATTERS 143
CHAPTER 12: CONCLUSION 149

FURTHER READING 159
ENDNOTES 161

INTRODUCTION

How can I justify writing yet another book about the National Health Service? Numerous books already exist and The Times Health Commission[1] had just published its important recommendations as I finished writing. It might be asked what I can add, but I am reassured that there is room for a contribution that focusses primarily on the needs of patients themselves and on the staff who care for them. That is where I begin, and my urge to write about it stems from the fact that I have spent my life working in the NHS or closely observing it and have always felt the need to extol it and its values.

I write from the perspective of an active clinician in an earlier life, a professor of medicine, a president of a medical royal college, and one who has closely observed how the NHS is managed and sometimes mismanaged. My experiences as a patient have been invaluable, too, and my role in scrutinising legislation in the House of Lords has also given me a little insight.

In writing about patients, it was impossible to ignore the fact that their health and well-being were dependent on so much more than the health services available to them, important though they may be. That led me to focus firstly on care in the community and social care. It is there where more attention on prevention and support is needed and where the dividends for individuals and society are potentially huge. That led me to devote my first chapter to this aspect of care. Secondly, it is clear that so much of adult physical and mental ill health is determined by social factors operating during childhood and adolescence. I cover some of this in the chapters on mental illness, maternity care, and public health. A major influence on the care patients receive when they are ill is the availability of caring medical, nursing, and other professionals. A discontented, disaffected, disillusioned, and constantly stressed workforce is not in the best position to provide the care that patients should expect. Caring for staff permeates chapters on social and primary care, and on secondary care.

In America in the 1960s, I was often asked why I wanted to return to the UK to 'socialised medicine', and I defended it to the hilt. It is because I still think it is worth defending that I feel the need to try to offer some ideas about how a service that is so sorely stretched might be rescued. I make no excuse, therefore, that this is a personal view of what I perceive might improve the lot of patients and those who care for them, and why I have tried to build on The Times Health Commission's recommendations. This is a different take on where the problems lie and what might be done about them.

There seems little doubt that there is widespread concern – right now – about the seeming failures in the provision of health care. The media are not slow to highlight its deficiencies. Barely a day goes by without a report of a cause for dismay.[2, 3, 4] But this picture of decline must be seen against the huge number of patients being dealt with; millions each year in primary care in the community and in hospitals, by dedicated staff working hard, often at the limits of their capacity.

Solutions on offer have too frequently depended on reorganising the structure and management of the service instead of focusing on – what I believe is more important –

the needs of patients. I have always believed that structure should follow function, not the other way around. It is from this end of the spectrum that I write; from the patients and their needs, leaving aside any structural manipulations. Some solutions do not need more funding and most certainly do not require any re-organisation of the management structure.

My aim is to explore in greater detail how patients are affected and how NHS staff are coping, or not, with a myriad of difficulties. It is here where we should be concentrating our efforts if we are to see the service regain a position of which we can be proud.

In the first chapter, I outline why the NHS was the envy of the world and how it remains a service, with its remarkable equity of access, free to everyone at the point of care, and why it is now fraying at the edges. Problems in primary care, care in the community and in hospitals dominate the news, and in the subsequent two chapters, I deal with the defects in social, community and primary care that have such a serious effect on patients. I discuss how and why the disaffection and demoralisation of the caring staff are having such an impact on the ways in which patients are treated. I go on to suggest some ways in which the most obvious problems may be eased.

In the next chapter, on care in hospitals, I point to where difficulties are arising. Correcting these serious problems requires attention to improving how frontline staff are treated and repairing the problems that arise from outside the hospitals. I discuss potential solutions to both of these issues. Mental health and maternity care services are special cases that deserve their own chapters. I deal with some of their well-publicised difficulties and discuss ways in which they might be mitigated.

Public Health comes next. This long-neglected service certainly suffers from underfunding by local authorities, but there are other systemic difficulties, too. Some of its problems go back much further than those that were exposed in the Government's response to the outbreak of Covid. And the public's health is determined by factors well outside the purview of the Department of Health, including transport, housing, unemployment, debt, and social deprivation. I discuss the reasons for its struggles and suggest ways in which they might be improved.

Research for new treatments and cures is vital for the future care of patients, and the UK has an enviable reputation in this field. But this, too, is now under threat, and in Chapter 9 I explain what the difficulties are and how they might be overcome.

I finish with chapters on some of the background to the positions we have reached in providing care in the UK. In the first, on trust and mistrust, I describe how damaging it is when the caring professions no longer trust the Government and vice versa. There is also a problem when the caring professions do not trust each other either. Regaining trust is no simple matter, but I offer some thoughts as to how it may be regained.

In the last two chapters, I discuss the multiple efforts by government in a series of Acts of Parliament to square the circle of providing a challenging and expensive service from strictly limited funds. A conundrum never easy to solve and one that remains unanswered. Finally, I discuss the ways in which health care is funded and tentatively offer one way in which we might approach it.

Rather than recommending another wholesale re-organisation of the service, I suggest how government money might be used to better effect, and how some defects may be overcome without recourse to more funds. There is only one reorganisation that I believe is worth considering, and it is where each of the limbs of the health services – social care, community and primary care, and secondary care – are unified. Sadly, this has proved impossible hitherto, and the idea that it might result from central government action is vanishingly small. I suggest that one way forward might be to increase support for local initiatives towards integration.

Overall, my intention is to explore what it is that we might do *now* that will allow the NHS and social care to recover and become services of which we can again be proud.

CHAPTER 1
THE ENVY OF THE WORLD?

One of the reasons the population is proud to be British is possession of the NHS. The way in which it was set up to provide health care without any restrictions on the ability to pay remains a concept that is worth protecting. It is why I do not go along with proposals to change the arrangement for funding to an insurance-based system.[5] Nor do I believe that privatisation, whatever that might mean, is acceptable. We would jettison the basic tenet of 'free at the point of service' at our peril. Since the NHS reached its 75th birthday in July 2023, and despite the many examples of excellent care, there have been calls for a complete reform of the way it is managed and funded.

One hears suggestions that the NHS is completely broken and that we should break it up entirely and start again with something new. I am not in that camp either. It's too trite and not thought through.

But that the NHS is in trouble is clear, and it is increasingly seen as symptomatic of Britain's general decline. It is 'the central symbol of what is wrong with Britain today.'[6]

As a nation, we seem to stumble from one crisis to another as we face the impact of Brexit, the Covid epidemic, and the invasion of Ukraine by Russia (with the subsequent inflation and energy problems that are increasing the cost of living). All of these distract governments and constrain their capacity to deal with the myriad difficulties facing the NHS. But we should not be deluded into believing that these recent pressures are the sole or even the main source of our difficulties. They had been building well before these recent problems.

Social and community care and the NHS have been in a slow, steady decline for many years. What is new is that the volume of complaints has been ratcheted up, and the recent strikes by health care professionals have simply served to emphasise the problems.

The size of the NHS is daunting, and the workload is huge. A million people attend general practice every day; that is almost 30 million attendees a month.[7] Hospitals deal with about 250,000 out-patients every day and carry out ten million operations a year. Almost 45,000 attend major Emergency Departments each day.[8] These are startling figures for a megalith service run as a single entity from central government. No surprise then that such large enterprises have proved extraordinarily difficult to manage or that they are failing.

What is remarkable is that despite these concerns, many in the population feel they are well cared for. But not everyone. The British Social Attitudes Survey found that only 29% of the population were completely satisfied with the service in 2022, a dramatic fall since 2010.[9, 10]

Reports of the problems faced by the population may be accurate but fail to describe the innumerable ways in which patients benefit every day from high-quality expert care for much of the time. Individually, many people feel enormous gratitude to their doctors, nurses, and carers. It is the overall picture of services under extreme stress where the population at large, and individuals within it, are under pressure. It is hardly doubted that services are failing and in more significant ways than ever before.

The challenges for any government to rescue the NHS are huge. Pledges by the Labour Party are well meant, and the Conservative Government's proposals are wordy, but both face huge barriers that will not be readily overcome. Both are constrained by limited resources and the difficulty of resolving the conflict inherent in devolving delivery of care while retaining responsibility on behalf of the taxpayer.

We have a long way to go as, for the first time in a century, since 2011, life expectancy has stopped rising.[11, 12] Not all due to a failing NHS, but it is clearly a contributing factor.

Too many patients are left drifting in a system ill-designed to meet their needs, and staff feel increasingly stressed as they recognise that – despite all their efforts – their NHS is failing to meet expectations.

The service has been designed around the needs of acutely ill patients who should be treated in hospital. That need should certainly be met, but it has been increasingly clear over several years that the much larger long-term needs of patients in the community have been sorely neglected. Patients with multiple morbidities, largely elderly, too often end up in hospital when their needs would be more suitably met within the community. It is primary care and, most obviously, social care that have been neglected in a damaging way. This is hardly a novel description of the current state of affairs. It has been the subject of repeated comments for years.[13, 14, 15, 16]

Numerous questions arise as to how and why the NHS and social care are failing so badly in so many ways. It is not as if we are short of reports, books, papers or Acts of Parliament to tell us that all is not well.

Health Ministers and Prime Ministers from the past have queued up with their ideas about how to rescue it, happily seeming to forget their own roles while in office and that they bore some responsibility for the current parlous position.

It has been a persistent struggle to provide a National Health Service within limited resources. But each of the reorganisations and re-reorganisations have focussed on the management and structure of the service. We now, in 2024, have returned from a multi-year unsuccessful flirtation with several models of an 'internal market' with a 'purchaser-provider split', to an 'integrated model' last fashionable in the 1970s and 1980s. This *La Ronde* has been an inordinately expensive and distracting exercise that has ultimately seen the service on its knees.

Certainly, more could be done with more money, and the need is starkly felt – especially in social care. But money is far from the only reason for our failing services. The Government must bear some of the blame because it cannot resist the pressure to change the administrative structure every few years. The caring professions, particularly the doctors, are in part responsible, too, because of their seemingly passive acceptance of government edicts and their apparent resistance to change. Both have caused difficulties, but governments must bear much of the responsibility.

Staffing Issues

It is the staff on the frontline – the doctors, nurses, physiotherapists and other ancillary staff, plus community care workers – that patients rely on, and who face many difficulties. Their lot is a demonstrably unhappy one.

The strikes of 2023/24 were just the tip of an iceberg of despair. They were not only about pay but an accumulating disenchantment with working conditions and an awareness that the services they provide are inadequate. The overarching problem for patients is that there are too few active staff, and those who are left feel disaffected and sometimes unsafe. Demoralised staff can lose their humanity, and there are reports of the disturbing brutalising of care.[17]

Government-inspired recruitment drives make too little impact, while efforts to retain staff remain poorly effective. There is a hole in the bucket as disaffected staff continue to leave. And it is by no means due to poor pay alone.

NHS and Social Care Divide

Providing care in the community, funded separately, is even less able than the NHS to keep up with demand and is extremely confusing for those in need who try to navigate it. The aging population is putting greater pressure on the services offered at the same time as these services are shrinking. This says nothing of the even larger but uncertain numbers of unpaid carers looking after disabled or family members at home.

There is also a serious discrepancy between the ways in which the NHS and social care are each funded and organised (Chapter 2). The NHS is provided by the state, free at the point of service and available for all. Social care is mostly funded through local authorities but provided by privately owned establishments. And it is means-tested. While private funding of health care in the UK accounts for only about 14% of the total, almost half the funding for community care is derived from individuals paying privately;

the remainder comes from local authorities. We thus have two distinct systems: a free health service and an almost entirely privately owned social care arrangement, means-tested, and subject to market forces with no national plan for the distribution and availability of its services. Little wonder then that, despite much brow-beating, a way in which these two disparate services may be integrated has proved so elusive.

Governments of different persuasions have, over the years, made much of the need for 'patient choice' and making the NHS more open to patients' wishes.[18] However, it has become clear that there are few if any options open for patients from which they can choose. Unless, of course, they choose to opt for private care. It is of interest that a survey of patients seeking private care revealed that many of them had tried to gain NHS treatment before doing so.[19] You might suspect that the NHS was failing in its efforts to offer choice despite the NHS Constitution enshrining patients' rights in law.

International comparisons

The UK lags behind most other OECD countries across many measures. We have higher mortality rates for cancer and other major diseases, fewer doctors, nurses, hospital beds and scanners, and the proportion of our GDP spent on health care per head of population is less than many.[20] The usual sense is that the health and social care services are underfunded for what is expected of them.[21, 22]

The NHS cost 7.3% of GDP in 2019-20; that is about 19% of total public expenditure, representing £164.1 billion. It had been about 7.0% to 7.4% of GDP for at least ten years before that. Seventy per cent of this expenditure is accounted for by salaries for the almost 1.4 million staff in the NHS.

In the EU, our neighbours spent rather more. The average day-to-day health spending in the UK between 2010 and 2019 was £3,005, which is 18% less than the EU14 average of £3,655.[21] If UK spending had matched the EU14 average, it would have been £227 billion per annum from 2010 to 2019, which is £40 billion more than the actual spend.[20]

Matching actual spend to that of France reveals a shortfall of about £40 billion, and compared with Germany a huge £73 billion shortfall, (a 21% and 39% difference in funding). In 2019-20, Germany spent 11.7% of GDP, France, 11.1%, Italy, 8.7%, Netherlands, 11.1%, Norway, 10.5%, Sweden, 10.8%, Canada, 11.0%, while the USA was off the scale at 16.7%.

Even though comparisons are not exact, as there are differences in how GDP is calculated, we have spent a smaller proportion of our wealth on health care than many similar democracies. And our total wealth is smaller. The event that markedly distorted these figures was the outbreak of Covid between 2019 and 2022. An explosion of untrammelled funding to control the epidemic in the UK resulted in a dramatic rise in NHS funding to £218.6 billion in 2020-21 and £216.8 in 2021-22 to be spent on emergency measures against Covid.[23] That is, 10.2% and 9.1% of GDP and about 20% of total public expenditure. Similar, if smaller, responses were seen in EU states. These remarkable increases were never likely to be sustained, and in 2022-23, spending was back down to £160.4 billion.

The situation in capital funding for buildings and estates is no better. If the UK had matched EU14 average capital investment, it would have funded 55% more cash than the £5.8 billion a year that the UK spent from 2010 to 2019.[21]

It is little comfort to know that most countries across Europe are now struggling with similar, if not as severe, problems. The adverse demography of ageing populations coupled with overworked medical and nursing staff are causing pressures in Germany, France, Italy and Spain.[23] Israel, long seen as an exemplar of health care, is suffering from shortages of medical and nursing staff and community carers.[24] Many medical staff in these countries are leaving their service, and fears are rising about the increasing costs of health care. Knowing that we are not alone does not help, but suggests that solutions will not be easy, will require very hard decisions, and will need to be shared by others. They will undoubtedly have to be based on a greater acceptance of the likely costs and sacrifices, and a determination to meet the challenges head-on.

Both the NHS and social care are huge enterprises, and that they are failing to keep up with demand is increasingly borne by everyone.

A discussion of the reasons why they are failing and the impact they are having on the population is an uncomfortable exercise. In the following chapters, I explore the issues we face and offer some suggestions as to how they might be tackled.

Summary

The founding principle of the NHS – that it is free, regardless of ability to pay – is well worth preserving. But despite many examples of excellent care, patient care is failing to meet the demands placed on it across the broad field of social and community care, primary care, and secondary care. The causes of failure are multiple and not all due to lack of funds, although that is certainly significant. Poorly motivated staff are too frequently unable to meet their patients' needs. Local authorities can barely afford to support care in the community, and the split between the NHS and social care damages efforts to encourage collaboration.

These are some of the issues that face patients today. They are the subject of more detailed examination in the following chapters.

I begin with how we provide care for the elderly and the needy in the community because it is here where – if we get it right – so many of the problems we face in the NHS are likely to be eased.

CHAPTER 2
SOCIAL CARE AND CARE IN THE COMMUNITY

The whole edifice of the NHS heavily depends on how we care for people in the community. Social care – provided in care homes and at home – overlaps with community care, including district nursing and children's services. But, the two most significant factors that have limited their effectiveness have been the lack of sufficient funding and completely disaffected care staff.

The Care Quality Commission Report of October 2023 – 'The state of health care and adult social care in England' – was damning about all services.[25] On social care, the authors wrote, somewhat mildly, 'Insufficient capacity in adult social care is continuing to contribute to delays in discharging people from hospital. Ongoing staffing and financial pressures in residential and community services are having an impact on the quality of people's care, with some at greater risk of not receiving the care they need.'[16]

Community and social care provide an unhappy picture of unmet demand and high unfilled staff numbers.

Demand

The figures are striking. Social care departments receive almost two million requests a year for help. (1.98 million in 2021/22, which equates to 5,420 requests every day of the year.[26])

Of these, about 30% are from disabled people below the age of 65, and the remainder from the more elderly. Some four out of five requests come from the community and not from hospitals. Despite only one in five coming from hospitals, it is there where all the publicity about inadequate services arises as they impinge directly on failures in the NHS. But it is the hidden majority that suffers the most.[27] It has been calculated that some 1.5 million people cannot get the care and support they need.[14, 28]

The history of the neglect of social care goes back a long way. The National Health Insurance Act of 1911 was an early attempt to support the elderly and infirm, but it was limited to the very poor. Before the start of the NHS in 1948, care for the elderly, the disabled, and the mentally ill, was hit and miss. But there were fewer elderly people then. Life expectancy was much shorter in 1948, at about 66 for men and 70 for women and – on average – we now live 13 years longer. The treatment of patients with mental illness was radically different when large numbers were incarcerated in huge mental hospitals. Many elderly and infirm were housed in long-stay geriatric wards and others in local authority, so-called 'Part III' accommodation. At the same time, a rather larger proportion was cared for at home at a time when a more cohesive and supportive family structure was the norm. Thus, although care in the community was not great, the pressures were much less. Nevertheless, and despite a lower demand, social and community care always seemed neglected as the poor relations of the NHS.

The National Health Service Act of 1948 saw local authorities being given responsibility for social care and care in the community in place of a range of charities and voluntary organisations. In the enthusiasm with which the new NHS was introduced, barely a thought was given to integrating it with social care. The NHS had enough to do with taking over 2,688 beds, 125,000 nurses and 5,000 specialist doctors. GPs were given a separate contract, and it was left to local authorities to deal with care in the community.

There was much to be done. The closing of large mental institutions and long-stay hospitals with the distribution of most residents to their homes and into smaller community care facilities was a huge and important task. 'Institutional' care was replaced by 'community' care. Undoubtedly, the residents benefitted, but concerns were immediately raised about whether the community was ready to receive or care for them. The availability of funds became the sticking point and has remained so.

Funding

It was soon recognised that neither the NHS nor local authorities were adequately funded as costs escalated way beyond original assumptions. It is the sad case that since that time, neither service has been seen as affordable. And worse has followed in social care as local authority funding has deteriorated. It has fallen by 55% as demands have increased. In effect this has caused a spending power reduction of 29%.[29]

Of local authority budgets, about half was spent on social care in 2010; in 2023, it was more like two-thirds, spent largely on the salaries of 1.6 million care staff.

Social care expenditure had remained fairly constant at around £17 to £18 billion per annum or about 0.9% of GDP. It rose temporarily in the Covid era to £22 billion in 2021-22, or 1.0% of GDP (2.1% of public expenditure).

At the same time, inflation has raised prices and demand has risen from an increasing number of vulnerable elderly. Requests for support are rising, too. Between 2015/16 and 2021/22, requests rose by 9%, from 1.81 to 1.98 million per annum.[30]

Although local authorities fund care for residents, they manage only about 4% of care homes themselves. And funding of care is the subject of much-agonised debate as the proportion to be paid by the residents themselves is a constant source of uncertainty.

Care homes are largely privately owned and run; some are small and independent, and others are part of large multi-site operations.

Needs of the Elderly

Demography is against social care provision. We are living longer, despite the recent flattening of life expectancy tables, and we are accumulating more disabilities that make us more needful of support.

In 2023, there were 11 million people aged over 65. A woman of 65 could expect to live 21 more years, while a man could expect 18.5 more years.[11]

Of those over 65 years of age, 3.3 million live alone, according to Age UK,[31] and it is recognised that loneliness is strongly associated with an increased mortality rate. They are vulnerable to falls, sleep deprivation, infections and depression, each of which hastens mortality in the elderly and infirm. Serious falls are three times more common in people in care homes than in their own homes, largely because they are likely to be an even more disabled group.

The figures hide the wide disparities in life expectancy between the most deprived 10% of the population and the least deprived 10%. A man in the South-East of England can expect to live until the age of 80.6 while a man in the North-East until just 77.6 years of age.[32]

A similar discrepancy is seen in women and the gap is even more stark when comparing the length of life lived free of disability. Disability-free life expectancy is clearly shorter in the North-East than in the South-East.[32] And the gradient of deprivation is getting steeper, while the burden of dementia grows heavier each year. Yet, local authority funding for social care – instead of responding to these differences by being higher in the most deprived areas – is, in fact, lower. The relationship between tax recovered by councils and average house price clearly demonstrates how deprived Northern areas are much worse off than affluent South-Eastern areas.[33]

Younger Persons' Needs

Most often, it is patients living alone with a disability (that makes it difficult for them to look after themselves) that pose a problem. It is not only elderly frail people but many younger disabled people of working age who also need help to enable them to get on with their lives. Bathing, dressing and preparing food may be beyond their abilities to manage themselves. They may need help with all of these, plus shopping and merely getting out of the house at times. Some are mentally disabled, while others have very complex medical needs. Above all, many are intensely lonely and need someone sympathetic with whom they can talk. Simple companionship and morale-boosting are part of the package of need. Then there are the particular and largely unmet needs of those with mental illness. Of these, patients with dementia pose a special problem. And their numbers are growing. With almost a million dementia sufferers in 2022, the numbers are set to rise over the next few years unless some treatment or, optimistically, a cure can be discovered.[34]

But how do local authorities fulfil responsibilities if they are starved of funds? Since 2022, the Care Quality Commission (CQC) has had a duty to ensure that high-quality care homes and carers are available to provide the full service. They, too, are likely to be hamstrung by the patchy distribution of privately owned care homes and by some uncertainty about what is to be included in a full package of care.

Care at Home

It is the case that most people in need are cared for at home by members of their family or close friends. Calculations by Age UK suggest that there are about five million such unpaid carers in the community.[35] Other calculations suggest that there may be twice that number of unpaid home carers, saving the exchequer some £162 billion per annum. That equates to about £445 million per day.

The fact that home carers have to make huge sacrifices – including the loss of jobs and earned income as well as personal freedom – is obvious, yet very few receive any financial support. Someone caring full-time at home for 35 hours a week can, if they are persistent, receive up to £76.75 per week. That's £2.20 per hour and only if their state pension is less than that.[35] For those with a severe enough disability, and who need care at home, carers can also receive an 'Attendance Allowance' of up to £101.75

per week if the person being cared-for needs assistance 24 hours a day. If they only need care during the day or during the night, they might receive the aforementioned £76.75 per week.[35]

Emma Duncan, writing in The Times,[36] describes the tortuous and prolonged process she needed, including completing a 30-page form, to gain an inadequate Attendance Allowance for her mother-in-law. Little wonder that only a small minority of home carers can manage the bureaucracy to gain any support.

The use of family and friends carers saves considerable costs to the taxpayer, but only at the expense of large numbers of loyal and compassionate people.

Slowly but surely, other types of support for care at home have been eroded. Home help, meals on wheels, district nurses and GP visits have all been radically pruned as staff numbers have declined. Community nurse numbers have fallen by 47% since 2009 and local authority-funded health visitor numbers by 30% during the same time.[37, 38] The smaller number of health visitors are distracted by a growing demand for child protection services, a particularly stressful responsibility.

Bureaucracy

Applicants for a care home place are faced with a daunting and confusing bureaucracy as they attempt to grapple with the system. Many do not know what support may be available to them and, too often, assume that they will not be entitled to anything.

Not surprisingly, applicants often face delays and obstruction. In March 2023, there were 434,243 people waiting for an assessment of their needs.[39] A third of those had waited for at least six months, and waiting lists are on the rise.

Others are caught in a service with poor communication, including, for example, between hospital and community services and between a myriad of disjointed care homes with multiple different owners. And general practitioners are too often outside the loop and not consulted by those assessing patients' needs. The criteria adopted for 'need' for social care are laid out in government regulations, but they are interpreted by local authorities who may or may not take account of any information from the applicants' GPs. No data on how the system is working are currently collected centrally, but one is left to assume it is fair.

If an applicant's need is approved, they then have to go through an assessment of whether or not they can afford to pay. This, again, involves much form-filling, and is often too difficult even for those in full possession of their senses. Their ability to pay is set at a level that severely limits access, and means-tested funding is a minefield. Anyone with assets worth more than £23,250 has to pay for all their care. If they own a home, and there can be few homes worth less than that, they pay for all their care.

That is not the end of it because if their assets are worth less than £23,250 but more than £14,250, they have to pay £1 per week for every £250 between the two limits. I hope that is clear! Governments since 2011 have found that the potential costs to the exchequer of social care were too high and hence unaffordable for the state. The Director of Age UK, Caroline Abraham, has written (in sorrow rather than anger) that anyone in need of care in the community right now struggles even more than in 2011. She wrote that 'budgets have failed to keep pace' and that '…the quality of care on offer is often pretty patchy … Social Care was at the tipping point and it is now clear that provision has broken down in some parts of the country.'[40]

So far as the NHS element of funding of social care is concerned, only some conditions will meet the criteria for help. For example, if a person has a cancer, then the NHS will cover the cost of community care, but not if someone has dementia or mental illness.

The limits placed on means testing have not been updated since 2010 and have not kept up with inflation or any other cost-of-living indicator. Even assets of less than £14,250 leave an applicant with the need to pay 'what they can afford from income only', whatever that means. The net result is that one in ten people over the age of 65 in care may be left with a bill of over £100,000 over the time they are in care.

Dilnot and Affordability

The Dilnot Report of 2011[41] proposed a way to ameliorate the problem. Dilnot's suggestion was that the maximum anyone should be liable to pay should be set at between £25,000 and £50,000 with a recommendation of £35,000.

Furthermore, the threshold beyond which self-payment should begin should be raised from £23,250 to £100,000. The cap on care costs prescribed by Dilnot were put into statute but never activated.

Now, 13 years on, we are still waiting for these recommendations to be put into effect. It's not that we have been short of many proposals for change; as we will see, it is just that none has borne fruit.

Local authority funding is made up of a government grant, local taxation including business rates income, and a modest grant from the NHS. Business rates incomes are lowest in the most deprived parts of the country where there are fewer large businesses. The remainder of care costs in care homes are covered by fees from individuals who self-pay.

This system is widely regarded as being inadequate. Numerous but unsuccessful efforts have been made by governments, not only in the UK, to try to repair it. Assessments of whether the costs of care in the community could be shared between clients and the state have often been made and found wanting in one way or another. It has always been the case that means testing has meant that anyone who could afford it paid for the total cost themselves. When Theresa May was Prime Minister in 2018, she proposed that costs should be shared and individuals who could afford it should pay for their residency and keep, either from their savings or by selling or renting their homes, while the state should cover their care costs. It was very unpopular, labelled as a 'dementia tax' and was widely held to be responsible for her loss of the premiership.

It was not the first time a scheme of this sort was suggested. In 1997, the then-new Labour Health Minister, Frank Dobson, decided to try to tackle this festering sore. He set up a Royal Commission under the chairmanship of Sir Stewart Sutherland (later Lord Sutherland) to examine the issue.[42] The report of the Commission, in 1999, recommended the splitting of responsibility for funding between the individual resident (who would pay for their accommodation) and the state (local authority) that would pay for care. The former was to be means-tested, and the latter free. But, two members of the Commission, Joel Joffe and David Lipsey (both later ennobled), felt that they could not support the proposal that the care provision segment should be free. They argued that it would rapidly become unaffordable and that it, too, should be means-tested, albeit with certain protections against people being forced to sell their homes.

Despite the plea for urgent action in the report, the minority view undoubtedly undermined its proposals. Perhaps more important was the fact that Frank Dobson, a strong supporter of the report, retired from the Department of Health to challenge for Mayor of London. None of his Labour successors in Health were interested. Part of the problem arose from the difficulty in discriminating between what were to be defined as care costs and what were residency and food costs.

There was one other potentially valuable proposal in that 1999 Royal Commission report that was for a new standing body – a National Care Commission – to bring together the various strands of long-term care under a single stewardship. Sadly, this was lost, too, and has not yet been resurrected.

Recent Government Proposals

More recently, the Conservative Government was pressed to respond to what was once again seen as a crisis. But the problem of how individuals would negotiate the two-stage assessment system – needs testing and means testing – has not been resolved. They are still dealt with separately and serially, thus taking up much frustrating time.

Promises made to bring forward a plan to reform the funding of social care during the Boris Johnson premiership were put off by the impact of Covid and have not been resurrected since. In September 2021, the Government published 'Build back better: Our plan for Health and Social Care' that included the aspiration to cap personal care costs, to assist those without substantial assets and provide wider support for 'the social care system'.

It aimed to provide £5.4 billion between 2022 and 2025, of which £1.7 billion would support 'system reform'. All this would be paid from a 1.25% levy on National Insurance contributions. A 'Health and Social Care Levy Act' placed it in statute in October 2021, but by September 2022, we were back to square one when the Government – under Liz Truss's premiership – delayed the additional funding. Later, Prime Minister Rishi Sunak reversed the levy in a new Act, the 'Health and Social Care (Repeal) Act'. The final blow came in the Chancellor's Autumn Statement of November 2022 when social care charging reforms were to be delayed for a further two years.

That has not been the end of reports and White Papers. We have had yet two more from the Government: 'People at the Heart of Care' (Adult Social Care Reform White Paper, December 2021)[43] and 'Next Steps to put People at the Heart of Care'.[44] Both were strong on ideas and avoided mention of the problems. They highlighted a lack of co-ordination and discontinuity of care, confusion in the ways care can be accessed, poor experiences and outcomes of care, and difficulties facing unpaid carers. Large sums of money were bandied about, £7.5 billion overall with £600 million to be released in 2023, according to an announcement in July that year. A new source – the Market Sustainability and Improvement Fund (MSIF) – was aimed at easing the transition, and the new Integrated Care

Systems and their Boards were to be responsible for ensuring the proper integration of services. It is disappointing to note that the purpose of the latter bodies was somewhat undermined by the failure to include representatives from the care sector in the membership of either of them. GP membership is apparently also facing difficulties.

More Funding Promises

After the two White Papers detailed above came a series of proposals for funded aspirations – to ensure everyone who needs it will 'receive outstanding quality and personalised support.'[43] They will be 'recognised as an individual with unique strengths and receive seamless health and social care from joined up services with everyone working together.'[44] In short, a vision of a nirvana as far as possible from current reality.

The National Audit Office pointed out that funding promises by government had not been fulfilled, and only some £700 million of the £1.7 billion remained for 2022-2025.[45] Further announcements in mid-2023 of an extra £600 million over two years just seemed to be the same as, if slightly less than, what was promised earlier. We are far from short of government plans, but we are desperately short of implementation. If ever there was a case for caution in accepting government funding proposals, look no further.

Care Homes

The transition to a care home service provided predominantly by private companies was gradual as the gap in public funding widened. In 1960, just 10% of community care homes were provided by private organisations; by

2020, it had risen to 83%. Now, only 4% is under local authority ownership and 13% under the voluntary sector. Government funding for social care rose by 5.7% per annum between 1997 and 2010, but since then it has fallen dramatically. It fell by 9.3% in real terms between 2010 and 2015. Little wonder it is struggling. While UK GDP has grown slowly, the proportion allowed for social care has remained constant at between 0.9% and 1.0% in each of the last ten years.

Progress has been limited by poor investment as the private sector has taken over much of the provision of care. The introduction of the internal market, heralded in the 1990 NHS and Community Care Act and enhanced in the 2012 Health and Social Care Act, focussed largely on the NHS, but it did much to encourage the direction of travel to market in social care.

The problem for those in need was exacerbated by the closure of 1,578 care homes between 2015 and 2020, when 48,600 residents found themselves in difficulties as they sought alternative accommodation, and the trends have continued.[46, 47] Many companies are vulnerable, and two very large ones, Southern Cross and Four Seasons Care, have become bankrupt since 2010. The Care Homes Association has calculated that the number of registered homes fell by about a third between 2019 and 2023, and as inflation bears down on profits, the total number of registered care homes continues to shrink; by a further 56 between January and May 2023 alone.

According to the King's Fund, the number of residential home places fell from 6.1 per every 100 people over 75 in 2012 to 4.8 in 2022.[48] The National Care Association attributed the fall to the rapid rise in costs with which care homes have to contend. Mortgage rates have risen, as have the costs of food and utilities, while funding from local authorities is restricted. That local authority funding is stretched to breaking point is clear.

The charge for an Authority-funded place should be a minimum of £900 per week, but they are often paid only between £600 and £700 per week.[49, 50] Some Authorities can afford even less and care home providers find themselves in serious financial difficulties. Increasingly, care homes are not seen as a valuable investment and private companies are by no means all making a profit. Just over 40% of clients, on average, pay for themselves privately. Until recently, care homes were not allowed to supplement their income by charging more to private clients than that paid for by local authorities. Many residents do now pay more.

Staff Problems

The great majority of the difficulties faced by people in need are directly the result of staffing deficiencies. These have been a constant factor for many years. Social care services employ more people than the NHS at 1.62 million, but turnover rates are extraordinarily high. At any one time, around 10% of posts are unfilled. Some 165,000 vacancies are advertised annually, and the fact that most of those leaving the service do so during their first 12 months speaks for an unhappy group of employees.[16, 51] High sickness and absentee rates make the staffing problems worse.

Social care workers' conditions of service would not be tolerated by any large employer keen to see a successful enterprise. They are at the bottom of the scale amongst health workers, neglected and under-appreciated. They do not yet have a nationally recognised and mandated training programme or qualification; they are not registered as those with professional qualifications and have virtually no prospect of career progression. A more enlightened scheme operates in Scotland where Scottish Social Care administers a mandatory registration programme of trained care workers. A similar scheme is operated in Wales by Social Care Wales. England lags behind, and we are only just waking up to the fact that English care workers need something similar. And, since the 1st of April, 2023, they have been paid at marginally above the national minimum wage rate at £10.42 per hour, while some 24% of care workers are on 'zero-hours' contracts.[51] Not much hope of a pension for them and no union to help them with their negotiations. Little wonder that they do not stay when they can earn more in any number of menial jobs in supermarkets and cafes.

There are suggestions, too, that care workers from overseas are being exploited by immoral intermediaries.[52]

The reason why so many do stay is because they feel they are doing a vitally important job for the good of their residents. In other words, the service is cashing in on the goodwill of those staff who continue working in it despite the unhappy combination of poor conditions and poor pay.

The Government's Papers of 2021 and 2023 made much of the need to offer greater support to care workers. The wish list included the desire for care staff to feel that social care is 'a rewarding career with clear opportunities to develop and progress, and where I feel valued,' and that 'they feel recognised for the important role they play; feel recognised for their skills; that there is a culture in their work place that supports their health and well-being; and that they are able to work effectively with professionals from other organisations.'[44] Needless to say, these are far from the experiences of care workers now, and there is a long way to go before they have any hope of being achieved.

Approved training programmes, continuing professional development, transportable qualifications so that carers can move around the country with their qualifications, digital skills training and a supportive website were all suggested in the White Paper. What was missing was their registration as qualified professionals and, unsurprisingly, pay was not mentioned at all. But at least the Government's aspirational plans are pointing in the right direction, even if they are far from reaching the desirable end.

It remains to be seen how much of this can be put into practice and whether it will encourage staff to stay and to stop the haemorrhage. It is not possible to gain too much confidence from the jargon in the Government's report, 'a review of market shaping capability initiatives to identify gaps and what action could address them, to accelerate a universal strengthening of the role.'[44] Quite!

Many care workers arrive from abroad. One estimate suggests that 70,000 have done so, but there are likely to be many more. They are valuable assets and there are considerable dangers if this source is threatened. Yet this is what recent government proposals will do. In an effort to reduce immigration, they intend to raise the minimum income a sponsor must earn before a visa can be issued for a non-UK spouse or family member. Currently, this stands at £18,600 and the proposal is to raise it to £38,700 by 2025. That is more than doubling it to a level no new care worker can hope to earn. Under pressure, the Government lowered the limit temporarily to £29,000, but that is above what a care worker starting out can earn, too. Currently, the Shortage Occupation List produced by the Migration Advisory Committee includes care workers. It remains to be seen whether that will continue under the more stringent conditions for immigrants introduced in 2024. The impact of these threats on social care services could be serious and severe.

Proposals for Change

It is vital and urgent that we get a firm grip on what is needed to bring up standards of care in the community, in primary and social care, and NHS community care.

People living longer with multiple and complex medical conditions are struggling to gain the services they need and may not receive treatment in time to prevent their illnesses from becoming serious. They may end up needing hospital care that is both more expensive for the taxpayer and bad for their health.

Here are some ways in which we might be able to ameliorate this sad state of affairs.

It is obvious that not all elderly people have the same needs. Three groups, each requiring different types of support, can be distinguished, and their support should be tailored to what they may or may not need. The first category is elderly but healthy; they should be offered health promotion programmes. The second category, probably the majority, have minor disabilities that interfere with their daily life to a modest degree. They need the integrated care of several professionals so that they can continue to live at home and engage within their capacity in normal communal, and even working, life. The third category have significant difficulties that interfere with their ability to live a normal life without support. They should be fully supported to live a life with the dignity they deserve. Each requires a different approach.

The Active Elderly

The first group, the active elderly, should be encouraged to engage in more exercise, join clubs, and increase social interaction. Gyms should be encouraged to set aside a day a week specifically for the elderly. They are not simply for the young, and it could be a valuable PR image for commercial gyms.

Many elderly people already engage in this, but this is an aspect of life in which public health and GPs play a key role that requires more than general messages on posters in their surgeries. An active PR campaign and community support programmes should be mounted and volunteer groups engaged. There are many opportunities for exercise in dance clubs, cycling, rambling groups, and more. Ensuring that the elderly know that they exist and are encouraged to join in should be publicised widely. A sense of purpose is vitally important in maintaining mental health. Volunteering and social engagement are invaluable in reducing the impact of loneliness on well-being.

Moderately Impaired Elderly

Much of the needs of the second group, those with modest but continuing medical needs, are mainly dealt with in primary care with support for daily living at home. It is where home helps, district nurses and health visitors are often needed, and it is where funding – limited though it is – should be directed. Investment to increase the number of these vital staff would lead to better care at home and less need for expensive and damaging admissions to hospitals or care homes.

Most Needful Elderly

It is, however, the third group, those so disabled that they require more support at home or in a care or nursing home, that requires particular attention.

Here, I deal with four aspects: making care work an attractive employment option; relieving the burden on applicants seeking means-tested support; and improving support for home carers.

Caring for the Carers

It is the caring staff where we must first focus our efforts, and on their shoulders rests care in the community. Without their co-operation, the service is doomed, and the impact is already being felt in the NHS at large. Yet it is these staff who are badly treated in ways that would not be tolerated in any other major organisation aiming to be successful. We must repair the many sources of disaffection under which they suffer.

And it is not all about their miserable pay. Firstly, they do not have a single representative body able to offer them a nationally mandated training programme or qualification. There are several bodies that offer training and there are several others that offer representation. However, none are recognised by government or the public as acting for them in ways that the Medical Royal Colleges and the Royal College of Nursing do in providing nationally accepted training curricula. Nor is there any oversight of the regulation of training bodies such that the GMC, GDA, or the Nursing and Midwifery Council provide for the medical, dental and nursing professions. Furthermore, there is no union such as the BMA or RCN offering protection for their members.

Without a recognised programme of training leading to a qualification that is registered by an approved body, carers will continue to be under-appreciated and neglected.

That must change if we are to see any impact on the huge turnover of staff, the large number of staff vacancies, and the high sickness and absentee rates.

The Care Quality Commission is aware of what is needed. In their 2023 report, they 'continue to call for a national workforce strategy that raises the status of the adult social care workforce and ensures that career progression, pay and rewards attract and retain the right professional staff in the right numbers.'[53]

And there is the nub of the problem: carers are not regarded as fully qualified professionals. There is a glimmer of hope that we may be edging towards some solutions in the recent government proposals outlined in 'Next Steps to Put People at the Heart of Care. A Plan for Adult Social Care System Reform'.[44] It is, however, full of aspirations but little in the way of practical means to achieve them.

Here, I provide some initial suggestions as to how they might achieve those aspirations.

Two needs, apart from salary, should be met first. A regulatory body for care workers and a qualification after passing through an approved training programme. Carers would then gain the recognition they deserve for the vital work they perform. I fear that it will not be possible to avoid some bureaucracy, as it will only be feasible if some form of regulation is instituted. Professional qualification depends on regulation.

One way forward would be for a working party to be set up, perhaps under the aegis of the Department of Health, and chaired by a distinguished figure knowledgeable of, but independent from, the social care world.

A discussion could then begin with the Health and Care Professions Council (HCPC). This is the body that registers some 15 professions allied to medicine, including physiotherapists, radiographers, art therapists, clinical psychologists, and chiropodists. The Council sets standards, approves education and training programmes and ensures that professional titles and qualifications are protected by law. Any new regulatory body for care workers would have to be recognised by this Council, and hence its views should be sought about what requirements would need to be met before any new profession could be accepted. Much work would need to be done before any such position could be reached. Here is one possible set of steps that may be worth exploring. There may well be others.

The Working Party, with a small number of leading members of significant social care organisations, should gather information and views widely from the caring organisations and others before making their recommendations. Their task would be to develop the basis for a body acceptable for registration by the HCPC. This would have to include an agreed set of education and training programmes for all care workers, a programme of continuing professional development, the conditions for the issuance of certificates, and the legal requirements for a registrable body. It should also seek to make recommendations for the length of time people spend in each of a set of grades suitable for the career progression of trainees. The banding system used for nurses and others could be adopted for career and pay progression.

There is a very long list of organisations offering training for social care workers. Many are in the form of distance learning and online training. Programmes vary in length and many offer certificates, some of which rely on self-assessment questionnaires and the approval of employers. Thus, the outline content of training may already be available and could be of considerable value. Some of these bodies could readily be incorporated as providers of education and training once they are approved by the new regulatory body. The HCPC would expect no less, as indeed would the overarching body, the Professional Standards Authority, that ensures that all regulatory bodies for the medical disciplines are fit for purpose.

The development of a career structure in which trained care workers could move up a set of grades over a number of years would provide the minimum basis for a satisfying career. Moving away from the prospect of the currently portrayed 'dead-end' job would do much to raise morale and reduce job losses. Some links to nursing would be helpful, too. The most obvious link might be with the Nursing Associate grade in the NHS and the possibility of a suitably qualified care worker having access to that type of career is likely to be attractive to recruits.

None of the above ideas are likely to be entirely novel to leaders in the field. The suggestions would clearly have to be acceptable to the many care workers' associations and those directly involved. I simply present them for discussion.

But the problem of poor pay remains formidable. Here, I will only hint at what an acceptable rate of pay might be. However, the current average rate set at about the minimal living wage by government does not do justice to the important roles care workers are expected to fulfil. A pay rate similar to, and sometimes less than, that received by those in menial and less stressful jobs is not an attractive proposition for recruits to care work. Rates at about Band 3 might be appropriate, though, and I discuss later where any additional funding might be gained.

Barriers to Those Seeking Support

Next, we need to deal with the many hurdles that those applying for care support must overcome. The strict limits placed by the means test for those applying for support before entering a care home allow few capable of passing them. The complex set of limits on means testing has not been uplifted with inflation since they were set many years ago. The Dilnot Report of 2011 proposed an increase in the cap over which applicants would have to pay.

Now is the time when something akin to the Dilnot proposals of 2011 should be activated, and achieved without recourse to further legislation. It would increase the cap beyond which applicants have to pay and reduce the total amount for which they are responsible during their lifetime. It is, however, worth considering the order of priorities for funding by local authorities. Relief for the means testing of individuals funding their care should be a second-order priority compared with funding for care staff and their support. After all, means testing relief is appreciated much more in affluent than in deprived regions of the country, while improved services affect all.

Ways in which the increased funding required by government can be provided are discussed later but immediate relief could be granted by reducing the time taken for assessment of claims for support and by taking an axe to the complex set of bureaucratic barriers that applicants must overcome. Reducing the paperwork might have the added benefit of saving clerical workers' time.

NHS Funding of Community Care

There is a further source of government support that can be gained from the NHS. Seriously ill patients with multiple health needs are entitled to free NHS care at home or in a care or nursing home. It is termed 'NHS Continuing Healthcare'. Unlike other support, it is not means tested and personal assets of any value are not taken into account. But those simply with old age and frailty do not qualify; only those with an illness accepted as a 'primary health need'.

Problems arise because few understand that this source of support is available and because of the postcode lottery involved in local Integrated Care Boards assessments. There is a strong case for a re-assessment of the ways in which this fund is made available. It certainly should be publicised to those for whom it might be relevant. Once again, minimising bureaucracy would be much appreciated by those in need.

Care at Home

On a similar theme, the ludicrously low pay achieved by the very few carers looking after the disabled at home should be radically overhauled. Currently, anyone providing 35 hours of care per week – and many have had to give up jobs to take this on – is entitled to £76.75 per week. That is £2.20 per hour. And to gain this pitiful recompense for saving the country the costs of a care home or hospital bed, applicants face bureaucratic hurdles involving form filling and much delay. This, too, should be the subject of further review to reduce the barriers faced by applicants and a more realistic and affordable award be calculated.

A National Care Commission

There is one other aspect that deserves mention and that is the proposal in the Sutherland Report of 1999 for a 'National Care Commission'. A standing agency or authority whose prime role would be to ensure continuing attention is given by government to the unmet needs of care in the community. I strongly commend this proposal.

The Times Health Care Commission recommends the establishment of a National Care System offering support in the community, administered locally and provided by a mixture of public and private providers. That certainly seems a valuable proposal but might be subject to considerable variability across the country. That is where a national body, such as a standing arm's length agency, akin to the National Care Commission mentioned above, could set standards and ensure that regional discrepancies are minimised.

Summary

The NHS is heavily dependent on a well-functioning social and community care sector. Yet, these systems are barely coping with the increasing demand from the elderly and disabled in the community. Three types of problem meet those in need, starting with the burdensome bureaucracy and the many delays faced by applicants for care that leave most frustrated and in limbo. A complicated assessment of need, followed by a stringent test of financial means, are too difficult for many to see their way through.

The second difficulty arises from the lack of enough care workers in homes and in the community. The high vacancy and turnover rates and the too frequent sickness and absenteeism speak for poor pay and an unsatisfying career for care workers.

The third area of concern is the poor support available to the many who care for relatives or friends at home.

Correcting these defects requires a stringent reduction in the bureaucracy faced by applicants and greater support for those engaged in support at home. With limited resources, local authorities have to prioritise their use of funds and any increases should be applied first to enhancing the care provided by care staff. This should include the introduction of recognised qualifications for care workers, leading to registration as professionals and a satisfying career structure.

Of importance, and next on the list, is a return to the Dilnot proposals of 2011 to reduce the financial burden on applicants for care. The proposal by the Times Health Commission to introduce a locally provided National Care System should be supplemented by a national agency such as a 'National Care Commission' to oversee and monitor these developments.

CHAPTER 3
PRIMARY CARE

Appointment Problems

Anecdotes about the failings in general practice fill the media but do not necessarily give a balanced picture of the huge number of daily interactions between doctors and patients – most of whom are satisfied. Typical was the front-page headline in The Times, 'Rise of the Month Long Wait Just to See Your G.P.'[2] The newspaper had discovered that the number of patients waiting more than 28 days to see their GP had risen to 14.9 million; that is 1 in 17 patients. It admitted that many other patients were seen on the same day and that those waiting longer may have had less serious issues, but the overall picture was depressing.

Primary care has come in for much criticism, too, especially since the outbreak of Covid, as patients complain that it is too difficult for them to get an appointment. If they are lucky, they may be offered a telephone consultation, but even then, it may be several days or weeks away. Reports of more than a million patients waiting to see their GP were published in 2023, and rural areas were worst off. Although 44% were seen on the same day, that left 56% of patients waiting longer, a discrepancy that has been difficult for too many to accept.

Simply phoning for an appointment can be problematic. It is a general rule that such calls should be made at a certain time, usually between 8-00 and 8-30 a.m., and there always seems to be a queue of callers. On average, the first hour on Mondays sees over 100 calls in a typical practice. Some practices allow appointments to be made in advance, but not all, and some patients are asked to phone again on the day for a follow-up consultation. Only some 10% of practices allow future follow-up appointments to be made.[54]

It is a problem that affects the elderly in particular. In July 2023, Age UK drew attention to the huge number of elderly patients attending Emergency Departments because they could not get a GP appointment; almost 700,000 in 2020.[31]

The number of patients seeking care is rising while the number of GPs is falling. On average, the number of GPs per 1,000 patients was 0.52 in 2015; by 2023, it was down to 0.44. Now, each GP has an average of 2,270 patients to care for, while it was 1,835 in 2015.[7]

There is little doubt that general practice is failing badly in too many parts of the UK, and general practitioners know it and regret it. They are frustrated and feel the heavy weight of knowing that they are failing. I have to admit that my own GP may be an exception. He practises a high standard of medicine and is accessible when needed.

But we have reached a situation where too many patients are unhappy with their GPs, and GPs are unhappy with the job they are doing.[55] GPs can hardly help knowing that they are not coping; they are sick and tired of the abuse they are receiving and are retiring early. Too many young doctors look to more interesting opportunities in Australia and New Zealand.

Rising Workloads

A few basic facts give a picture of a service under stress.

The number of consultations by GPs is steadily rising. Some 370 million consultations in 2021, a rise of 18.5%

compared with 2019. This rise was accompanied by a fall in GP numbers of 5% during the previous five years.

There were 36,467 GPs in post in the NHS in 2023. More than 70% of them worked part-time so full-time equivalence was much lower at 27,231, according to the Royal College of General Practitioners.[56] The majority, some 58%, were women. An average GP cares for 10% more patients than in 2015.

Bureaucracy

General practitioners are also distracted by an overwhelming bureaucracy. Non-clinical administrative tasks have risen by over a quarter since 2019 alone. And, for many, time spent chasing up laboratory and other investigation reports and making appointments are administrative tasks that should rightly be undertaken by other staff but who are often unavailable. Each week, GPs must deal with over 100 reports of laboratory results and letters and emails from consultants and others. Often, they take this load home to deal with, quietly away from the telephone. Dr Kate Fallon, a GP, told the Commons Select Committee on 'The Future of General Practice' that 'I have a list on my toolbar with all the blood results that have come in from all the patients, letters that have come in from consultants, discharge letters and anyone else who wants to write to us, which all has to be looked at and put into the patient record. There are other things like insurance reports, DVLA reports and that sort of thing. ... Prescriptions? It is 60 to 100 [per day]. Blood results? Again 60 to 100 [per day]. Letters? It is 20 to 30 a day. Maybe two or three reports a week.'[57]

Many GPs sit on committees that help regulate or oversee the service. Clinical Commissioning Groups (CCGs), (now Integrated Care Boards and, until very recently, Local Medical Committees, amongst others) take up far too much time for those leading the profession. Those contracting with the NHS for their services, manage their own businesses. That alone poses an extra management load, often performed out of hours. Managing their practice and responding to regulatory bodies takes up almost 30% of their time, leaving less for direct patient care. One GP told me that it took up 50% of her time away from direct patient care. Little wonder that GPs complain about this increasing load of administrative tasks.

The demand from increasing numbers of patients, the distractions of non-clinical work, and the fall in staff availability is making life all but impossible for many.

We now have a vicious circle of GPs failing to cope with the demand placed on them, followed by a strong desire to retire from the frontline well before their retirement age, thus adding to the shortage of practitioners.

Only about 50% of new GP trainees take up full-time employment. Many now opt for a 'portfolio' career to maintain their sanity.[55] They work two days a week in their practice, for example, and perhaps a couple of days in their local hospital, then engage in a research proposal or social activities for a further day. This work pattern has considerable advantages. It improves morale and helps the NHS, but it diminishes the capacity of primary care to provide its prime function.[56]

There are problems for nurses in primary care, too. The attractiveness of nursing in general practice is diminished when it is recognised that they lose much in transferring from the NHS. They lose maternity pay, sick pay, and study day release because they are not part of the NHS. Some practices make up this deficit, but by no means all do.

The advent of Covid clearly exacerbated the problems of primary care, but they were building well before that extra stress. Little wonder that we are seeing a growth of private general practice, modest as yet, but following the lines of dentistry where it is almost impossible to be seen by an NHS dentist in many parts of the country. Unsurprising, too, that patients turn to dialling 111 for help and/or arrive unannounced at busy Emergency Departments in hospitals. The problems are not aided by poorer recruitment as young doctors seek better opportunities elsewhere, often now in Australia or New Zealand.[58, 59] In those countries, too, staff shortages have encouraged a recruitment drive that clearly includes more inducements than our own.

Changing Work Patterns and Continuity of Care

The new GP contract of 2004 saw marked changes in primary care. Methods of remuneration were altered, GPs increasingly worked in larger groups, and out-of-hours responsibilities dropped remarkably. Now, very few GPs engage in home visits. They have too little time from all their other responsibilities, and they remember that they were sometimes called out for trivial complaints.

Two other aspects have also been damaged. The first is the loss of continuity of care. In a busy practice, it is the unusual patient who manages to see the same doctor at each visit. This matters little for patients with a single and relatively minor complaint, but the loss of continuity is problematic for those with long-term conditions in need of close monitoring by a doctor who knows them well.

New ways of accessing services are supposed to reduce the demand on GPs. Dialling 111, walk-in centres, online and telephone consultations – they each have a supportive role, but patients are rightly persistent in wanting to talk directly to their doctor. Nor has the promise held out by self-help apps – such as 'GP at Hand' – or the use of algorithms for self-diagnosis, proved entirely fruitful.

Data derived from GP contacts and from 111 calls fed by the 'Policy Exchange' through the 'NHS Gateway' into a symptom-checker app was supposed to provide accurate information for doctors and patients. In the USA and the UK, algorithms derived from huge banks of clinical data have been used to analyse patients' symptoms and proven diagnostically superior to doctors in some circumstances. Where the problems lie is in ensuring that the data going *into* the analyses are accurate; some have been shown to be unreliable. The management of patients based on the interpretation of the results of such automated analysis may be faulty, and the doctor will always be turned to for help in understanding the results of the analysis. Confusion is not helped by the number of different apps that are becoming available.[60]

Sadly, these systems have not always taken account of the vagaries of symptoms of patients with multiple diseases. The place of AI could assist GPs and their patients, but the inference that it will somehow lessen the load on GPs seems unfounded. At the end of the day, patients need to consult their doctor, as they will always require a 'second opinion'.

Only some 38% of patients in England felt that they had any relationship with their GP, yet continuity of care matters. That seems to be supported by data from Norway, where it is the norm for patients to be followed up by the same doctor. There, sickness and mortality rates have responded well. However, other factors may operate in Norway, not least the fact that GPs look after only some 1,200 patients compared with the average of about 2,270 in Britain.

New modes of investigation and treatment are keeping patients alive and well for longer but pose challenges to practitioners as they try to keep up with demand and new knowledge.

These are the factors that contribute to the loss of GPs.[61] The average age of retirement is 59.6 years, and the total numbers have gone down by 7% since 2016. When asked, over 40% of GPs said that they would retire within the following five years. Much more worrying is the loss of over one in five GPs under the age of 30 who left in 2022.[58]

The Government is making a well-trumpeted effort to increase the numbers in practice by raising recruitment and medical student numbers, but it will have a difficult job to keep up with the current rate of loss. The prediction by the Health Foundation that there will be a shortfall of some 8,800 GPs by 2030 gives little comfort that current workforce plans will be entirely effective.[62]

Workforce planning is fraught with difficulties, and using broad figures for doctors is far too inexact. Account has not always been taken of the fact that an increasing number of doctors will only work part-time and retire before the age of 60 years. Maternity and paternity leave in a young workforce and a desire to care for children for longer will only dilute the number of active practitioners.

A desire to have a comfortable work-life balance is not restricted to GPs. It is common across many professions, but it has the unfortunate consequence of reducing the number of working staff and increasing the pressure on those carrying the load.

The problems are widely felt but they are particularly acute in practices with few doctors that do not have the resources or the flexibility to deal with the workload. The loss of one member of staff due to illness, maternity leave, or retirement may make a small practice unviable.

More Pressures and The Impact of Social Deprivation

Eight hundred practices have closed since 2013, some by joining forces with others, but many lost forever.[63] Brighton has seen eight out of its 36 practices close since 2015.[64]

The mismatch between health needs and GP numbers is particularly felt in deprived areas of the country. Hull, for example, has a significantly higher deprivation score than the average across England, with high unemployment rates and more cancer and coronary heart disease. Yet it also had the highest number of patients per GP at 2,804, according to data from the Nuffield Trust.[65] These disparities are reflected in higher mortality rates where resources are least available and where North/South divides are most in evidence.

Larger group practices can cope if run efficiently, but they, too, are vulnerable as pressures grow. The demand for efficiency and effectiveness is keenly felt, and only the best practices manage it well. Spreading good practice has proved inordinately difficult and, as we will see, depends not only on the goodwill and involvement of a disillusioned profession but rather more on government support. After many years of delay and much expense and obfuscation, the introduction of electronic medical records has been taken up by most GPs and hospitals. But not everywhere, and patients themselves are too often unable to gain access to their test results and consultant opinions. GPs remain wary about the possibility of leaks of confidential data about their patients. This is particularly the case if the data are to be used in research.

The complexity of GPs' workloads has increased substantially. At the same time, their ability to change and innovate has been constrained by the rigid and inflexible control under which they operate. I was told that some no longer feel safe as the medico-legal risks increase. New requirements seem to be thrust upon them from above – too often – with little regard for the time that is needed for them to be put into practice.

There are too many regulatory bodies assessing every aspect of their work, yet the data that are collected do not seem to be used for any discernible purpose. One GP told me that it is in the lower rungs of management that a culture of 'no' permeates the system and where clerks are given responsibility for dealing with the work of GPs. Too much time is spent in meetings at which decisions are unusual. 'If we got rid of 2/3 of ICB activities, no one would notice,' said one GP.

Problems with Referrals to Secondary Care

Just as the hospital service is overwhelmed by patients who feel they should be cared for in primary care, GPs feel that hospitals are loading more and more responsibilities onto their shoulders. Referrals to consultants are restricted by the 'E-Referral System' under 'Advice and Guidance' that require patients to have blood tests and X-rays before referral, all adding to delays. This system took the place of the disliked 'Choose and Book' system, or the 'Lose and Book' system as it became known. GPs are asked to take on a range of further responsibilities after discharge from hospital, including post-surgical care, prescriptions, and follow-up care, often with modest information.

Proposals for Change

From all the above descriptions, it is clear that there are too few active GPs to meet the demand placed upon them and that they and their patients are suffering. There is a desperate need to make improvements, and there are some indications as to how this might be achieved.

Lessening the administrative load, improving managerial efficiency, and increasing the ability to innovate are all aims that require action.

Each practice should be given the support staff they need to take some of the administrative work off GPs' shoulders. One example could be to build upon the 'Additional Roles Staff' budget that funds each Primary Care Network for what is known as 'social prescribing'; that is, help for patients with non-clinical needs such as housing, finance and employment. It is the case that this budget is underspent, and since non-clinical needs are often met by the Citizens Advice Bureau and a range of charitable organisations, this funding should be diverted to primary care practices. They could certainly use help with administrative responsibilities.

Writing sick notes takes up too much time, too, and could be devolved to occupational health services.

In turn, there is a need to improve IT systems in primary care, and although costs may not be large, persuading ICBs and local authorities to help with funding has not been easy. Decisions such as these should be moved up beyond the obstructions of clerks and others in the lower echelons of the ICBs. While improvement in IT systems is important, the place of AI tools in primary care is not yet proven. More research in this rapidly developing field is due. Its full potential is awaited, and much interesting speculation about its impact on practice is now common. A lot will depend on proven reliability.

That rapid decisions for action can be made was clearly demonstrated during the Covid outbreak when the mobilisation of GPs in the vaccination programme was successfully achieved. This culture for rapid action to reach efficient decisions should be spread throughout the activities of ICBs. Boards should now examine how they might achieve this end.

Single-handed GPs are much rarer than they were a few years ago, and the move to larger practices has continued apace, especially in large conurbations. It may have impaired continuity of care as patients meet a different doctor at each visit, but it does not have to be like that, and steps can and should be taken to obviate it.

The recent introduction of associate physicians is potentially useful, if controversial. Partially trained in a shorter time, they have been shown to be helpful sitting halfway between fully-trained nurses and doctors. Suspected by the medical profession at large, and the public, they have nevertheless clearly shown themselves to be an invaluable part of the team in which the GP is always available. Patients have been favourably impressed by the care of knowledgeable assistant doctors who give them more time. Gaining the confidence of medical staff and patients will now be an important step.

There are savings to be made through premises and the use of support staff in larger groups. The 'polyclinics' suggested by Lord Darzi in his review of the NHS[66] have morphed into the recently proposed 'Community Diagnostic Centres' where large practices incorporate a range of diagnostic facilities such as X-rays, breast screening, echocardiography, and diabetic eye screening, as well as physiotherapy and occupational therapy. Such buildings exist in a few places and successfully provide patients with an efficient one-stop service. There is room to build more of them, especially in large conurbations, although they may not be so feasible in country areas with widespread populations.

There is some controversy about whether GPs should continue to be self-employed or become employees of the NHS. Although it might seem tidier, the evidence that it would improve the service to patients is unclear. Some GPs find that they are relieved of the managerial responsibilities associated with owning their business. Others might look over their shoulders at the level of disenchantment within their NHS colleagues and feel they are better off where they are. My main interest is in patient care, and I will not become distracted by this area of controversy.

It is clear that patient care would be improved if GPs had more time for their clinical work. The possibility that GPs can be persuaded to work in their practice for an average of one more day per week – from, say, three to four days – could make a significant difference to the availability of services. It would require government-inspired incentives but is a worthwhile aim. Appointments would be sped up, and the continuity of care would improve. But GPs must be relieved of the overwhelming administrative jobs they do, of attending innumerable fruitless meetings, and they must be supported by agile managers capable of rapid action when the need arises. Under these conditions, recruitment into primary care may be increased and professionals might be persuaded to remain in the service until normal retirement age. Certainly, increasing medical student numbers will be necessary, but it is the attention we give now to making general practice an attractive proposition that will make the biggest impact on patient care.

Summary

Reports of long delays for appointments for patients to see their GP are far too common. As the number of requests to see a GP has increased, the number of GPs has fallen. Continuity of care is threatened. Administrative tasks take up far too much time away from clinical care. The workload of GPs has increased, resulting in a stressed, unhappy set of doctors, many of whom retire early.

To improve primary care, the load of non-clinical bureaucracy must be relieved. The IT systems available to GPs usually function well, but too many are unfit for purpose and do not link to other parts of the service. Investment here would be invaluable. The further development of Community Diagnostic Centres offers advantages in conurbations of a reasonable size. The role of AI in primary care offers potential advantages but will require careful evaluation before wide introduction. Encouragement and support from the ICBs for greater freedoms for GPs to innovate could bear dividends.

Above all, there is a desperate need to increase the number of GPs by enhancing *retention*. Attention to their non-clinical workload and conditions of service could help, and incentives to lengthen the average clinical week from three to four days (where appropriate) should be debated.

CHAPTER 4
CARE IN HOSPITAL

Problems arising in hospital care are too often secondary to defects in social and primary care. Resolution of those will certainly help. But not everything will be perfect, and many of the difficulties faced by secondary care require corrective action within the service itself.

There are currently (as of December 2023) 7.2 million patients on waiting lists for hospital admission in England and Wales. The Government has been quick to announce the triumphant reduction from 7.7 million in September.

Waiting Lists

Waiting lists would not be a problem if patients were not waiting long, but almost 360,000 have been waiting for a year or more, and many more have been waiting between 6 and 12 months. Ministers boast that the number of patients waiting more than 18 months has been reduced by 90%, but the attempt by government to reach the pitifully unambitious target of no patients waiting for 18 months or more by April 2023 has failed.[67]

There were still over 10,000 patients waiting more than 18 months by then. Efforts have been made to speed up referrals for cancer patients, but the 62-day target has been missed, and over 19,000 such patients are waiting longer to start treatment.[68]

It is, however, largely patients with non-acute conditions, such as cataracts or painful and disabling arthritic knees or hips, that are left waiting much longer. Even when admitted, there are too many sad stories of operations being cancelled and patients sent home. And it may happen more than once for some patients because of the pressures from emergency admissions. In turn, the strikes of nurses and doctors in 2023 saw thousands of operations and appointments cancelled. Continuing strikes by trainee doctors into 2024 point to even longer lists and waiting times. Of course, there is wide variation amongst hospitals and not all (nor everywhere) are failing to keep up. But far too many are.

Emergency Departments

Patients sitting or lying in Accident and Emergency Departments – for hours or even days – speak for an emergency service that is inadequate to meet the demands placed on it. Age UK reported that a third of patients attending Accident and Emergency Departments were over 75 years old, largely because they had been unable to see their GP.[69]

Less than two-thirds of all patients were dealt with within four hours, according to the latest figures (2023). The Government had a target of 95% being managed within four hours but had to lower it to 76% when it was clear that the higher target could not be reached. The figure of 61% that is now being achieved is clearly well below the latest target.[70] For those being admitted, a wait of more than 12 hours is the norm.[71] And long waits in Emergency Departments can be dangerous. A study of over five million patients revealed an increase in all-cause mortality associated with delays in admission. Mortality rates were 8% higher for those waiting more than six hours from arrival at the Emergency Department.[72] Little wonder that the Government dislikes targets.

Several factors contribute to this sorry state of affairs. Limited access to general practitioners prompts many to use hospital Emergency Departments as their first port of call. Even if they phone 111, as advised, they are too frequently told to attend a hospital by staff that lean towards caution. The net result is that far too many patients crowd into Emergency Departments when they, and the hospital, would be much better off if they were cared for in the community. Seriously ill patients may be left on trolleys, sometimes in corridors, as they wait to be admitted. Their hold-up is due to the lack of available beds to which they can be admitted. Over 95% bed occupancy rates leave little or no room for manoeuvre. And it is not just a 'winter pressure' problem; it is now year-round.

Too many beds are occupied by patients waiting to be discharged. About 15% of inpatients are ready and keen to go home, but there is no-one to care for them either in their own homes or in care homes. And the numbers are rising. About 14,000 patients fitted into this category in 2022-23 compared with 4,500 in 2018-19.[30] These are patients, usually elderly and in need of temporary or long-term support as they recover from a disabling stroke or fractured hip, for example. It is the lack of care in the community that is a major cause of the backlog in hospitals. And the problem is confounded by one in six elderly patients having to be re-admitted within 30 days, again speaking of inadequacies in primary and social care. Queues of ambulances outside hospitals waiting to discharge their patients into an over-extended Emergency Department are too common.

Medical and nursing staff work under a pressure that is increasingly intolerable in Emergency Departments. They are fully aware that they are not meeting their patients' needs. They are completely disheartened when they are obliged to explain to patients, yet again, why their operation has been cancelled or why they are lying in discomfort for hours in the Emergency Department waiting for a bed. They are too often exhausted as they rush from patient to patient in inadequately staffed departments. Sickness and absenteeism rates are high. Expensive temporary agency staff are called in too frequently, and they are not always aware of local arrangements as they search around for equipment and support.

This is the picture of an Emergency Department crowded with confused patients simply waiting for something to happen to them while frustrated staff rush around, too busy to stop and care. Not everywhere, and not all the time, but too frequently to give any comfort.

It is clear that to improve patient care in hospitals, we have to look outside hospitals first. It is in primary care and care in the community where glaring deficiencies have a direct impact on the capacity of hospitals to deliver. It is here where the prevention of admissions and the speedy, efficient discharge of patients will have the most significant effect. But it is also how hospital staff, and not only doctors and nurses, are treated that impinges directly on the care of patients.

Staffing Matters

As with social care staff, it is with hospital staff and how to correct their obvious disenchantment with the service that we should focus on. Doctors and nurses are the obvious target here, but others involved in care – the physiotherapists, midwives, and radiographers – cannot be ignored.

"Well-run companies can operate only with the consent of their workforce. Well-run bosses run companies well with the consent of their workforce." (Lord Offord of Garvel, Hansard, December 19th, 2023).

Any large, successful company understands the value of an engaged and contented workforce. It will know that if its employees feel supported, they are likely to be more productive and proactive, have less absenteeism, and lower sickness rates. They will generally stay in employment for longer, and turnover rates will be low. Sadly, this is far from the case in NHS hospitals. In Richard Layard's book, 'Happiness', he clearly lays out the factors that underlie successful enterprises.[73] A contented and appreciated workforce is demonstrably more productive than one which feels neglected and disheartened.

The anger and frustration that spilled over into the strikes by nurses and doctors in 2023 are much more than simply about pay. Pay is just the latest manifestation of a festering frustration.

The extent of the unhappiness was clearly demonstrated in the 2022 NHS Staff Survey.[74] Over 600,000 employees responded, and while the nurses formed the largest group, most employee types were represented. It was hardly surprising that only 25.6% were satisfied with their level of pay, but that was clearly not their only concern. Almost 43% would not recommend their organisation as a place to work, and 37% were unhappy with the standards of care provided for them. Some 58% were not satisfied that their organisation valued their work. Worryingly, 9% experienced discrimination at work.

Thirty-eight percent said they could not speak up about their concerns, and over 50% were not confident that anyone would listen to their concerns even if they expressed them. Only slightly fewer thought that their concerns about clinical care were likely to be heeded (43%).

The same sad story emerged when they were asked whether they had any control and influence. Only 53.7% felt they had a choice about how to do their work, and almost 50% said that they were not involved in decisions about changes. Almost the same proportion felt they were unable to make improvements happen. In other words, they felt alienated from helping the service to improve.

Their workload was widely regarded as too heavy. 57% found that they were unable to meet all their conflicting demands, and some 76% experienced unrealistic time pressures. About 15% had received physical abuse from patients or their relatives, and 11.1% had been bullied or abused by their managers.

Given this background, it was not surprising that about 45% had felt unwell with work-related stress and 34% felt burnt-out by their work. A high proportion were exhausted by the thought of another day at work, only about half looked forward to going to work, and a third were unenthusiastic about their jobs. Only about half of respondents felt that they had a good work-life balance. A set of questions about team-working revealed that 30% or more were not enamoured by the opportunities available and, in some instances, this was worsening. Almost 75%

indicated that there was not enough staff available to do the work.

Perhaps most depressing of all was the fact that almost a third (32.3%) said that they often thought about leaving their organisation, and 17.3% said they would leave as soon as they could find another job. Vacancy rates for doctors in 2023 were about 8,500, while for nurses, it was 40,000.

These sad data simply emphasise the fact that the NHS is not a happy place in which to work. Daniel Chandler, in his book, 'Free and Equal', writes that the NHS workplace is 'a sphere of subservience and powerlessness quite unlike any other domain of life in a modern democracy.'[75]

It is not simply that staff are rushed and under pressure – although that is the result of understaffing, absenteeism, and high sickness rates – but the fact that they feel under-appreciated. Their views are hardly ever sought, they are told what to do by managers who are not always sympathetic, and there is little respect given for what they do. Or at least, that is how they perceive it. Too often, directives from on high, made in committees they do not know, pile in on them, and they simply have to comply without fully understanding *why*. Little wonder that they feel that they are being treated as cogs in the wheel rather than the professionals they are.

The managers, too, are simply responding to a tune to which they are required to dance. They are dominated by a need to keep to a strict budget and are rewarded for their financial control and by trying to cope with the numbers of patients being dealt with, less so for the standard of their service to patients. They are inundated with regulatory demands that leave little room for innovation, and unless they are built of a particularly strong character, they just pass on the instructions they are given to their staff. They receive several visits a year from various regulatory bodies to check on their activities so that they scarcely have time to even think about innovation. Running a large hospital is no simple matter, but the heavy pressure from without and the day-to-day issues within lead to burn-out. Chief executives only remain in office for an average of three years before they move on. That is nowhere near enough time for them to make a sufficient mark that can lead to continuing improvement in care.

Teamworking

The team spirit that characterised working relations in hospital care in the last half of the 20th century has been slowly but surely eroded. Nurses and doctors worked closely together. Ward rounds where every patient was fully discussed by the team are no longer the norm. If a consultant goes to see her patients now, she is lucky if a nurse accompanies her. If she is so fortunate, it is unlikely to be the same nurse each time and rarely the most senior nurse. Instructions about treating patients are usually written notes and less often through verbal discussion. Junior doctors are even less likely to have the presence of a nurse to help them as they consider the management of a patient.

The division between nurses and doctors can only be damaging for patient care. The root causes of the rift go back a long way, and they crept up on both the nursing and medical professions with scarcely a murmur of dissent.

A cohesive spirit and good working relations were common when nurses lived in nurses' homes and doctors were resident in the hospital. Now, most nurses and doctors are no longer resident and live separately in their own homes. Of course, it has the advantage of allowing staff to live independent lives and to cohabit with their partners, but something has been lost. Not only can it be expensive for individuals, but it also limits the social cohesion of those who work in hospitals.

Staff restaurants and the doctors' mess have disappeared and only general cafes for visitors are available. There are few restaurants, cafes or cafeterias open after 6-00 pm and none after 7-00 pm in any hospital I have contacted. Staff working overnight have access only to slot machine dispensers. Thus, there is nowhere for doctors and nurses to meet regularly to arrange easy referrals. Discussion about patients between professionals is no longer fostered, and precious time is lost in efforts to write or phone colleagues. Just another symptom of poor support as social and professional interaction is no longer readily obtained. Adding to the sense of disenchantment by staff are the car parking charges that nurses and doctors have to pay along with visitors. Few hospitals provide free parking for staff and parking charges pose a burden that some may not be able to afford.

Nurses

For nurses, it was the changes to their career structure and education that improved standards but had some unpredicted, adverse effects on patient care and teamwork.

The Salmon Report of 1966 and the Briggs Report of 1972 introduced them to a formal career structure in which they could rise through a series of grades beyond the ward sister level. Then, starting with Project 2000 during the

1990s, nursing education became increasingly formalised, and by 2009 nurses were required to gain a university qualification. Standards of nursing were undoubtedly enhanced as they now became increasingly capable of highly specialised care with considerable expertise in a range of medical disciplines. Oncology, cardiology, gastroenterology and surgical nurses, for example, are now experts in their fields and offer high standards of care.

However, two unhelpful consequences emerged,

The new career structure ensured that a nurse in charge of a ward of patients, a sister or charge nurse, was no longer in a long-term career post. She or he was on a ladder upon which there were several more steps they could climb. And as higher rungs beckoned, they moved on every couple of years. The old-style, long-serving sister was replaced by a succession of younger staff, sometimes lacking the ability to exert their authority. Wards of patients and the doctors involved in their care could no longer rely as heavily as they used to on a sister who knew what it was to bear the ultimate responsibility for the care of patients in her charge. The new, highly-educated and undoubtedly competent nurse in charge is occupied with managing her ward through her computer and collating data for reports she is impelled to compile. Within a relatively short time, she is ready to move on up the grades beyond the ward level. Continuity and authority at the critical ward level have been impaired.

Dr H A Dewar wrote as early as 1978, '…one wonders whether any nurse with ability and self-respect will ever consent to remain a ward sister for more than a short term. She will hold the lowest job but one in this hierarchy, and she will have above her a nursing officer who is fully equipped to act with the maximum power of detailed interference but who, because she has five wards to 'control', will neither take the doctor's instructions directly nor have the patients' confidence.'[76] Now, 35 years later, his predictions remain unhappily unchanged.

The development of a structured career for nurses with progression through the grades has improved the management of nursing, but not necessarily basic care for patients.

And, with the high educational standards of nurses, a gap has appeared. A lack of those interested in careers that purely require basic nursing skills has opened up. Care of sick patients in general medical wards requires not only attention to the treatment of their diseases but also involves ensuring that they are fed, bathed, and turned, and that their toilet needs are met. Above all, a friendly and familiar face to whom patients can turn for support in their time of maximum vulnerability. This was often covered by those in the now defunct State Enrolled Nursing (SEN) grade, and more recently the role has been taken on by Nursing Associates or Nursing Auxiliaries. These grades have not yet proved sufficiently popular and career prospects in the grades are not attractive. There are signs, too, that a career in nursing may be losing its allure. Applications for nurse training courses have fallen,[77] the drop-out rate is said to be 13%, and three out of five do not enter NHS employment after qualifying.[78]

Fully qualified nurses are as caring and supportive as anyone could wish for, but too often, they are in a rush and constantly changing. A fresh face every shift simply confuses patients unsure whether details of their care have been passed on. And once they reach the grade of ward sister, their thoughts are distracted by further career prospects.

It is these changes in nursing that were intended with the best of motives — to meet the need for a highly-educated and competent profession — that have also allowed these negative effects to emerge.

I suggest, later, how changes might be made to improve the issues I have described.

Doctors

Nurse training is not the only aspect of professional change that has impinged negatively on patients and their attendants. For these, we need to focus on the medical profession.

The post-graduate training of doctors has gone through a series of changes, some of which have been within the control of the profession. As a minor example, it is disheartening that the profession has allowed itself to agree to label trainee doctors by numbers and not names. It smacks of the Gulag when first-year trainees are now FY1s and second-years are FY2s. Trainees then move on to become ST1s and on up to ST6s at around the age of 32 to 34 years before obtaining a consultant post. ST4s to ST6s are the old-style senior registrars but are now demeaned by their labels. I have not heard many complaints about this numbering system, but I cannot imagine it gives much comfort or confidence to patients to be introduced to an ST4 doctor.

That, however, is not the least of what has been lost and worse came with the advent of EU regulations several years ago. Two elements conspired to inflict uncertainty on patient care; the march to standardise and regulate postgraduate training across the EU, plus the EU working time directive.

Long hours of work for junior doctors were sometimes unbearable, and burn-out too frequent. To try to correct this, the European Working Time Directive made it illegal for doctors to work more than 48 hours per week. That this caused more difficulties than it solved soon became clear. There were too few doctors to cover the whole 24 hours of the day that was required. Imaginative rota schemes were developed, and the margins of the 48 hours soon became eroded as doctors found that they could not quit in the middle of operations or interviews with patients. Experience gained from continuity of care was precious for patients and doctors alike, and many of the latter found themselves working unofficially at the ends of shifts. Simply being 'on-call', perhaps asleep in bed, was also counted as part of the 48 hours as negotiated by the BMA, so the Directive was often ignored.

Another problem arose when training became splintered by the rotation system. Consultants involved in teaching found that trainees were constantly on the move in their four-month rotations through a range of experiences. Training became threatened as exposure between individual trainees and trainers was curtailed.

Continuity of care, as well as training, came under greater threat with the new schemes brought in as a result of an EU edict to standardise training across Europe. It was aimed to ease cross-EU border movement of staff, a laudable aim but one that was fraught with problems for the NHS. Firstly, immigrant doctors from other EU countries had simply to demonstrate that they had spent the requisite number of years in training in their specialty. There was no requirement for the content of their training or the competences that they had achieved to be checked. Indeed, UK authorities were specifically prevented from assessing these attributes. The General Medical Council, and the hastily set up Specialist Training Authority (STA), had to rely only on whether immigrant doctors had spent the required number of years in training but not the content of that training. Only later did it become possible for the GMC even to assess competence in the English language; it was never given responsibility for assessing clinical competence. It gives me no comfort to remember that I struggled hard but unsuccessfully while I was Chair of the STA to change the UK system to a more helpful EU Directive that was available. This would have allowed us to assess the competences of EU doctors applying to practise in the UK just as we can for trainees from non-EU countries such as America and Australia. It was the medical profession that proved more resistant than government on this occasion. Clinical competence can still not be assessed before interview for employment of EU graduates in the NHS. Perhaps BREXIT opens an opportunity to change this?

It was the impact on the training of UK specialist doctors that became immediately clear. A set number of years of training was accepted, and these were usually shorter than had been the previous norm. More had to be packed in, with relatively short-term rotations through a range of experiences. It eventually settled down, but the need for trainees to stop work – sometimes part-way through a learning experience because of the end of their shift – was unhelpful.

It was this combination of splintering of training programmes and the time-limited rotas of trainees because of the working-time directive, coupled with the demise of the doctors' mess and loss of a residency for trainee doctors, that all constrained teamworking and continuity of care. Patients in hospital were faced with a bewildering series of different doctors rotating through their training programmes and on short-term rotas. The only constant became the consultant in charge, but she or he was not always on the ward or immediately available. They had other commitments, for example in the outpatient clinics and operating theatres.

Communication between consultants and their junior staff was now constrained, as with the nurses on the ward. Too often, consultants found themselves seeing their inpatients without junior staff or nurses and communication about care was breaking down. Not much has improved since then, and while it is possible to see well-functioning teams here and there, they are only achieved by extremely dedicated and imaginative doctors and nurses working hard to overcome the constraints under which they work.

The recent government fanfare announcing significant increases in the recruitment of doctors will eventually relieve some of the pressures, but unless the underlying loss of morale and the factors contributing to it are addressed, we will continue to see a haemorrhaging of staff. Pouring staff in at the top while losing them at almost the same rate at the bottom is grossly inefficient. And patients suffer. It is a common experience for a patient in a hospital bed to feel confused and neglected. He or she meets a different doctor or nurse each day or even more frequently as staff rotate through their shifts. Continuity of care has been lost and patients' treatment is compromised. This is the experience of far too many patients, but few complain as they leave hospital feeling grateful to have survived!

Beds and Physical Resources

Tackling waiting lists inevitably entails attention to the availability of beds and facilities, and it is not helped by the reduction in acute hospital bed numbers from 180,000 in 1987 to 141,000 in 2019. Much of the reduction has been warranted by improved surgical techniques and the increasing use of day surgery. But now we have gone too far. The UK has 2.5 beds per 1,000 of the population while the average across a bundle of Western countries is 3.2.[20]

Too many hospitals are in a poor state of repair, and there is a backlog of work to be done on them. This is not helped by the recently discovered problems due to eroding and unsafe types of concrete used to build them in the 1950s and 60s. Promises of 40 new hospitals to be built by 2030 by Prime Minister Boris Johnson have been shown to be unachievable, and we remain with a shortage of hospital beds compared with most civilised countries.

Improved surgical practice has reduced the need for beds, but the question now is *how many* beds do we need? If, for example, the 15% of beds currently occupied by patients who should not be there became available, then the shortfall would be much less. Much depends, therefore, on supporting care in the community rather than simply building more hospitals. That, at least, is the testable argument that can be made. Meanwhile, the shortage of beds is biting hard. In late 2023, the Government announced the introduction of 'surgical hubs' (where operating theatres and staff are solely dedicated to treating 'cold' waiting list patients) to enable surgeons to be able to operate unencumbered by acute emergency admissions.[79] Trials had shown that such a system could allow the rapid turnover of patients currently on long waiting lists – requiring hip operations, for example, or cataract surgery. Spreading this example is good in principle but depends entirely on the availability of surgeons, anaesthetists, nurses, porters and other support staff.[80] They are not standing around waiting, and there will still be a need for surgeons and other staff to deal with emergencies, including elderly patients with fractured hips and those with traumatic injuries. But separating 'cold' surgery from the day-to-day need to cope with 'emergencies' is a move in the right direction if we can face up to the need for sufficient staff. Spreading that practice where it can be achieved is clearly worthwhile.

The purchase of care for NHS patients from the private sector has helped relieve acute shortages, but it can only be a short-term measure. Longer-term, it is likely to be expensive.

Scanners

Underinvestment has also led to the UK having the lowest number of CT and MRI scanners per million people at 16.1 compared, for example, with France at 33.6, Ireland at 36.4, and Germany at 69.8.[20]

Efforts to obviate a shortage of MRI and CT scanners by using those that are available in the evenings and weekends is a worthy aim but, again, it is the availability of radiographers and radiologists that is the rate-limiting step. The loss of many radiographers from Europe following Brexit is proving difficult to repair but the increasing use of

AI to interpret scans may come to the rescue of shortages of radiologists.

Whatever palliative measures are adopted, however, it will prove difficult to make up for the discrepancy between the availability of scanners in the UK and similar countries in Europe. We clearly lag behind here – as in many other areas – and greater investment in scanners and staff will produce dividends in improved care. The detection of early disease would follow, cancer cure rates would rise to match other countries, and savings would follow in the NHS.

IT and AI

Artificial intelligence (AI) is being promoted by the Government as a valuable aid to the Health Service. It will, they suggest, increase its efficiency and thereby reduce its costs.

It is worth teasing out exactly where AI may prove valuable for patients and where it is unlikely to help. It is increasingly evident that it will be invaluable in the research leading to new drugs. Using sophisticated genetic analytic tools, drugs can be designed specifically to attack disease variants. Pharmaceutical companies are using AI to short-circuit the time taken to examine large numbers of molecular structure variations. Google DeepMind has a drug discovery spin-off (Isomorphic Labs) that, they suggest, will reduce the drug discovery stage from five years to two years. Others will no doubt follow. These developments will improve the search for new treatments for future patients but not immediately for current patients. It seems likely that AI will also assist in the interpretation of laboratory and imaging results, thus speeding the process, and doctors and patients will have access to their results much more quickly. Greater uncertainty exists in its potential to improve the clinical care that comes from the doctor-patient relationship.

Proposals for Change

Nurses

I recognise that it would be easy for me to step on the toes of a profession for which I have enormous respect. Nursing is an increasingly complex role, requiring highly-trained and skilled professionals, and it is full of dedicated, well-qualified individuals. It is well recognised that they are paid at a level that is not commensurate with their responsibilities and the level of risk they are managing.[81] They are university-educated, and many go on to highly specialised care with considerable expertise.

But I hope that they accept that there are some aspects of nursing that deserve comment and that I write from the position of a keen admirer of the ways in which they fulfil their roles so effectively.

The first unanticipated problem arose from the changes in the career and pay structure that left the nurse in charge of a ward of patients on a transient rung of a ladder, leading out of direct patient contact. Pay structures now value management roles more than clinical roles, encouraging nurses to move on and away from direct patient care. However, the ward sister or charge nurse is the key post as far as patients are concerned. They expect this nurse to be sufficiently mature and authoritative and in whom they can place their trust. And we are in danger that she or he will not receive the respect of patients, doctors, or other nurses. That contrasts with fond memories, not always accurate, of the regard in which old-fashioned ward sisters were held.

Here, I suggest that the post of the nursing sister or charge nurse responsible for a ward should be made a more permanent career-grade position, akin to that of consultant doctors who have reached the end of their training. If nursing sisters are to be encouraged to remain in that post for more than two or three years, they should be given access to the higher grades to which they would aspire as if they had moved up the career ladder off the ward. And of course, they should be paid at the relevant rate.[81]

A higher-graded post and a commensurate salary would make ward responsibility a more attractive option. In the past, I have suggested that the salary should be in line with that of consultant doctors to recognise the high level of responsibility for patients that the post entails, but I recognise that this could create many difficulties in nursing pay across all grades. Nevertheless, it is an indicator of the esteem to which a nurse in charge of a ward of patients should be held, as against posts in more administrative roles. None of this can be achieved without the full support of the nursing profession itself, but I do hope that The Royal College of Nursing will give the proposal, with its aim of improving patient care, careful consideration.

There is one other aspect of nursing that deserves attention, and that is the gap left in care by the loss of State Enrolled Nursing posts (SENs). The move to a university-educated workforce has offered clear benefits in raising educational standards and improving care.[82] Nurses are now highly qualified, they have improved mortality rates, and they are capable of doing so much more for patients than was previously the case. They are certainly as caring and effective at providing patients with emotional and other nursing support as ever, but they may be distracted by the specialisms opening up to them. Nurses may not remain content if their role is simply to help patients with their feeding, bathing, pain relief, and emotional support. This is a gap that can be filled by the relatively new nursing auxiliaries or nursing associates. Recruitment to these posts is just as important as government efforts to recruit more nurses, but they seem to have slipped behind in the greater publicity given to nurse recruitment. Neither of these new posts requires a university education and will appeal to many who wish to care for patients with less pressure to enter higher education. The Government should now encourage more applications to posts for which more generalist practice is needed.

My two proposals – enhancing the role of the ward sister and increasing the recruitment of nursing associates and nursing assistants – may help improve the care of patients in hospitals. However, instilling a sense that *all* nurses are appreciated for the vital work they perform is essential, and we are a long way from persuading the Government and the NHS that they should be taking this seriously.

Doctors

The discontent amongst doctors reached boiling point in 2023 and early 2024 with prolonged strikes. But even if the matter of pay is resolved, it will be extremely difficult to repair the myriad sources of discontent that have been building over many years.

It is here where much effort should be focussed to bring back the ethos that provided a more satisfying career with patients at the centre. Consultants certainly feel strongly that the service has lost most of the attractive features of the career they remember, perhaps through rose-tinted spectacles. Those in training have never known them. Those halcyon days were never perfect, and in any case, it is not now feasible to think of going back to them. But an effort to recapture the more valuable features should be considered. The most obvious loss has been the team spirit that permeated medical and nursing practice. That the team working together was a valuable way of providing patient care is hardly doubted. Instead of a bewildering series of staff paying them fleeting attention, patients knew who their doctors were, and could rely on a constant nurse in charge of their care. Continuity of care is now hard to sustain.

Is it possible to return to some elements of teamworking? A start could be made by the medical profession itself taking a grip on the 'ward round'. A consultant should ensure that her trainees are available at a specified time, several times a week, to accompany her during discussions with all her patients. It can and should be insisted upon. A senior nurse should be present throughout. Discussion could start in a side room so that all concerned with the care of their patients will have all the information they require and can share it with the team. This already happens in several hospitals, but the practice should now be spread. The 'ward round', where the team sees every patient, provides an opportunity for patients, doctors, and nurses to each understand the care needed and being given. Removing misinformation and misunderstandings can only be helped by everyone having the same full picture. It is not always easy to gather staff together for such an exercise. Trainee doctor rotas and nursing distractions pull in other directions and it requires persistence and some authority to make it work. But an effort should now be made to recapture the team ward round.

What must change, too, is the disenchantment that is rife amongst doctors and nurses. They now have the sense that they are simply cogs in a wheel, driven by a distant government and its local administrative machinery. Any large, successful company will endorse the view that this must be changed. We should begin by re-introducing some semblance of democracy at the hospital level so that doctors and nurses feel that they are being heard as major contributors to the work of the hospital. The introduction of a Representative Committee for Doctors and Nurses in each hospital would be a first step. Acknowledging that such a development might have adverse consequences, safeguards must be introduced. To avoid setting up an adversarial system – with the staff on one side and the administration on the other – there should be a regular meeting between staff and managerial representatives. To obviate the antipathy of other types of staff, the possibility of representative sub-committees should also be explored. A chair should be elected, and an agenda should be set for each meeting to avoid descent into a free-for-all. Clinical leadership is vital and requires the selection and election of acceptable leading clinicians.

There are likely to be several other ways in which staff can be given the freedom to play their part and contribute to the ways in which their hospital is providing care. These are currently denied, and that situation must be repaired.

Trainee Doctors

Any idea that medical trainees are purely there to be trained and not to provide any service has been clearly dismissed by the enormous impact on all services by their strikes of 2023/24.

Large numbers of cancelled operations and outpatient clinics speak to a heavy service dependence on so-called 'junior' doctors. Yet their training needs dominate the ways they are employed. Short rotas of training through a variety of experiences may or may not provide valuable training, but they do little for continuity of care or for teamworking.

For early-year trainees (so-called F1s and F2s), consideration should now be given to whether four-month rotations are sufficient for training and experience. Four months is barely adequate for trainers and trainees to understand each other. An assessment should be made of whether six-month rotations would provide a better fit for both training and continuity, and this is something the Medical Royal Colleges should consider.

Then, there are the rota arrangements inflicted on the service by the EU Working Time Directive. There is a good case for this rigid and formulaic arrangement to be revisited. Trainees leaving at the end of a shift – part-way through dealing with their patients, as some may be tempted to do – is far from ideal. There might be an opportunity now we have left the EU to examine how well the rota system is working. Is it being flouted? Are trainees really being protected from overwork? Is their training helped or inhibited? And what impact is it having on the continuity of care for their patients? These are questions that need urgent attention. I suspect that the Colleges and Post-Graduate Deans will already be considering these questions, but there is now some urgency for them and the BMA to find answers.

There are many other ways to try to enhance team spirit and reduce disenchantment. Monthly meetings of consultant staff can bring all the specialties together; in the past, they provided valuable opportunities to meet colleagues to discuss their patients and issues of the day. They were a feature of the early years of the NHS that was discouraged by managers of hospital trusts. There seems no reason why they cannot be reinstituted, save for the excuse of lack of time. But given enough will by consultants, they are likely to be appreciated, and it is unlikely that the hospital administration would want to try to ban such meetings. It is one way of reducing unhelpful divisions and misunderstandings between clinicians and managers.

The net result of a more contented staff is a better deal for patients, greater productivity, less turnover, less absenteeism, and less early retirement. Surely, that is what the patients need, and it is what government should be aiming for.

Facilities

Much is made in the Times Health Commission about how modern technology will transform health and social care in the future. Certainly, it is an exciting prospect, but I must express a hint of scepticism. No doubt, it will influence some ways medicine is practised, but the question of whether the heavy load placed on services will be eased is not clear. I note the remarkable advances already achieved in medicine by the use, for example, of MRI and CT scanners, keyhole surgery, fibre optics, and coronary artery stenting, all heralded as invaluable advances in patient care, but they have not solved the problem of meeting all the needs of patients with limited funds. Care may or may not be transformed, but we should not expect to lessen the load or save any money.

There are suggestions that AI, with its facility to analyse huge banks of data derived from millions of patients, could assist in diagnosis. Its algorithms could rapidly spew out a diagnostic list, by likelihood, together with suggested treatments for any set of symptoms a patient may offer. The problem for patients is in interpreting all the data presented to them, and they will need to engage their doctors in understanding the results. Another problem is that some of the information currently entered into data banks may be inaccurate or distorted. That has already caused problems, and until the available algorithms can be made reliable, it would be wise to maintain a position of caution.

Whether AI will result in more accurate diagnosis, reduced confusion, or saved time remains to be seen. Meanwhile, these fascinating developments will need to be continually assessed.

However, AI has much more potential than in aiding the interpretation of scans and X-rays and in drug development. At the Sourasky Medical Center in Tel Aviv, Israel, for example, they have gone much further in digitally identifying patients by facial recognition as they enter 'self-triage booths' for blood pressure and temperature measurement. Robotic assistance helps as patients pass through the maze of its Emergency Department.

Much more relevant and productive is the progress that can come from improving the usage of Information Technology (IT). In the best hospitals and most general practices, it provides medical staff with ready access to patients' electronic records, including their test results, correspondence, and drug information. Patients can gain their repeat prescriptions and other helpful information online, too. And in excellent GP practices and hospitals, staff can bring up all the information necessary to help in their care wherever a patient is seen. But, sadly, it is not happening everywhere. Too many hospitals have yet to emerge from the disasters of some years ago when government efforts to introduce a uniform computerised system across the whole of the NHS failed miserably and very expensively. We now have several systems in place; unfortunately, they do not all speak to each other.

IT can work well and has been shown to be efficient and invaluable in some places. What is needed now is the spread of good practice to all hospitals and GP practices, and the Government should take steps to ensure that it happens. It should be possible for a doctor meeting a patient from any part of the country to have ready access to all that patient's records. Furthermore, the patients themselves should be able to have access to their own records. It was suggested that each patient could carry a 'credit card' sized memory drive on which all their clinical data can be downloaded. It is technically feasible but will probably be unnecessary when it is now feasible for patients to gain all they need to know on their smartphone or laptop. Currently, it is resisted by some in fear of patient confidentiality becoming vulnerable. It is unfortunate that some GPs are reluctant to allow their patients to have access to their own data when we know that it is the norm not only in many countries but also in many practices in the UK.

The Government should urgently make the cost-effective IT system that is already available in many hospitals and practices available in every place where patients are seen. There seems to be no good reason, either, why the system should not be available to district nurses working in the community. And none of this should be excessively expensive.

The use of remote monitoring of patients in 'virtual wards' has some potential once the infrastructure can be fully developed. Its success will depend on whether there will be enough staff to monitor patients being observed and whether they will be based in hospitals, primary care, or social care. That it can be done well has been demonstrated at Sheba Hospital in Israel, where hundreds of patients are monitored remotely. Sensors in the ceiling check wearable devices that record vital signs and whether patients have fallen. There is more work to do on a fascinating innovation in practice.

Staff Support

A dining room or canteen for staff in a hospital is an unusual phenomenon, yet it used to be a widely appreciated place to meet with colleagues. We should be pressing for its replacement. Furthermore, the availability of meals for staff working out of hours at night and at weekends should be the norm. Currently, the only access to food after 6-00 or 7-00 pm and at weekends in most hospitals is through dispensing machines. It is a disgrace; it does not reflect modern-day 24-hour working and should now be challenged.

With a captive population of hundreds or even thousands of staff, hospitals must be an attractive proposition for many catering companies. They should be encouraged to bring in restaurants or cafeterias specifically for staff. A reasonable chef might even attract staff and their partners to dine in the hospital. That may be too much to expect, but we should be encouraging managers to reconsider this and other ways of making their hospital an attractive place to work.

A further source of discontent is the charging for car parking that all hospital employees have to pay. Although the income may be a valuable subsidy to cash-strapped Trusts, they should consider the well-being of their staff in their calculations. Any employer trying to support their staff would do nothing less.

Summary

Many of the problems arising in hospital care are due to defects in primary, community, and social care, yet these services are managed and funded separately. While these divisions continue, their problems have to be dealt with separately, too.

Some of the solutions to long waiting lists, cancelled operations, and delayed discharges lie out with hospitals, but some problems require attention within.

Patient care is best provided where the caring professions work as teams. Sadly, this is no longer the norm, and efforts to reintroduce elements of teamwork should be strongly encouraged. Ward rounds at which doctors, trainees, and senior nurses all attend on a regular basis should be the aim. In this way, patients can gain the confidence that all of those engaged in their care are fully aware of every aspect of their case. Ward rounds should be formalised, and regular staff meetings should be reinstituted. More effective clinical leadership is required. Royal Colleges and Postgraduate Deans should pay attention to the question of whether current disruptive training programmes are achieving their aims.

Nursing career structures should be re-examined, and the nursing sister in charge of a ward should be given greater authority and a career in charge of a ward, together with appropriate pay rewards. Nursing associate and auxiliary posts should be given greater prominence and reward to fill a gap in the needs of patients.

Repairs to hospitals' physical estates are urgently needed, but it is the staffing difficulties described here that require even more effort. Greater appreciation of all staff by the provision of catering after hours is essential. Cold slot machine food for staff working at night is unacceptable.

CHAPTER 5
MENTAL HEALTH SERVICES

The incidence of mental illness, especially anxiety and depression, is rising in the general adult population and over three million people access treatment each year.[83] Pressures following Covid, Brexit, and the impact of the Ukrainian war are causing costs of living, levels of debt, and unemployment to rise. They weigh heavily and have increased the number of people seeking help for their mental ill health. Demand is now outstripping supply in many parts of the country. And the incidence is highest in areas of deprivation.[83]

Talking Therapies

The most successful form of therapy for anxiety and depression is 'NHS Talking Therapy' (previously known as the inelegant 'Improving Access to Psychological Therapies' (IAPT). More than half of patients going through a six-week course of talking therapy, usually as CBT (Cognitive Behaviour Therapy), show such improvement that they can return to normal activities, including work.[84] Another 20% gain some improvement. It is an extremely cost-effective treatment and does not involve taking drugs. The problem is that this service is not readily available everywhere. Waiting times for access to this treatment vary between four days in the best areas to almost 20 weeks in the worst, mostly in areas of deprivation.[83] Ten areas of England are not meeting the six-week target for people to be seen.

Talking therapies are given largely by clinical psychologists, and in 2023, there was a 12% vacancy rate, and over half of Mental Health Trusts (57%) reported staff shortages. This, coupled with the high vacancy rates for mental health nurses, means that a very effective type of care that can convert sick people into productive workers is being seriously hampered (see Layard[85]). A very short-sighted approach.

Mental illness is a huge drain on the resources not only to individual sufferers but also to the exchequer.[83] If ever there was a case for improving the care of patients with anxiety and depression, it is emphasised by the fact that they are responsible for the largest proportion of claimants for disability and sickness benefits. The costs of these benefits are rising alarmingly as the number of claimants is rising. The total claim in 2023 was £32.5 billion and is forecast to rise.[84] There are now 40,000 claimants per month through the Personal Independence Payment (PIP) system; the cost of mental health problems is about 36% of payments.[86, 87]

There is another large group of individuals who suffer from addiction to alcohol, or drugs, or even gambling who could be treated and returned to work given enough staff to treat them. People with personality disorders leading to self-harm or anti-social behaviour are disruptive but could be helped if psychological therapies were available for them. Too often, the availability of care is abysmally small, yet the successful management of patients can improve their lives and their capacity to engage in work.[85]

Treatment of Psychosis

More serious types of mental illnesses pose different sets of problems. Psychotic behaviour – due to a variety of causes – affects some 1.5 to 3.5% of the population. The main outcome is a loss of contact with reality and includes delusions, hallucinations, and disorganised thought and behaviour. Schizophrenia, affecting about 15 people per 100,000 of the population, is but one obvious cause. Substance abuse, brain injury, and severe infections can cause psychotic episodes. Anorexia nervosa, although less common, has the highest death rate.[88] Many of these patients need urgent attention, and crisis teams are there – in theory – to provide rapid support. Sadly, only about a third of such patients are seen within the recommended four hours. 'Mind' reported that demand was outstripping supply with a 10% rise in patients using mental health services.[89] Sixteen thousand adults and 20,000 children were not able to access care, with wide variation across the country. Over 40% of Mental Health Trusts report a shortage of staff. There is a 20% vacancy rate for adult mental health nurses. With one in five staff vacancies, it is not an attractive career for many.

Community mental health care is lacking, and too many patients end up in acute hospitals as emergencies. Mental health hospitals are running at over 95% capacity, and they can barely cope with the burden of patients needing inpatient care. Mental Health Trusts are using a growing list of private mental health inpatient services such that the private sector provides 30% of inpatient care at a cost of over £13 million per month. The Government promised more funding for mental health care, but this has been swallowed up by inflation and increasing demand.

It is the case that there are some patients detained in hospitals for prolonged periods who should not be there. This is true of those with autism and learning difficulties. The long-awaited Mental Health Bill promises to correct this, but it has disappeared off the screen.

Patients who are at risk of suicide or who have attempted it are most often admitted to general medical wards. It is there, too, where patients with dementia who need care are being admitted.

Staff working under such stressful conditions sometimes leads to high-profile reports of poor care and abuse of patients.

The Public Accounts Committee, in July 2023, noted a rise in the number of staff leaving mental health services and attributed it in part to a fall in morale and a lack of self-esteem.[90] Psychiatric consultants are in short supply, too, with a vacancy rate of some 10% in adult psychiatry.

Child and Adolescent Psychiatry

The situation with childhood psychiatry is no better. A significant proportion of children persistently absent from school have Attention Deficit Hyperactive Disorder (ADHD), yet the services available for their assessment and management vary widely across the regions. In some areas, children are seen within 12 weeks; in others – Northern Ireland, for example – it is several years. The National Autistic Society (NAS) has drawn attention to the more than two thousand people with autism or learning disabilities who are being held, quite wrongly, in mental health hospitals.[91] It has been described as a 'human rights crisis' by Tim Nicholls of the NAS.

Rachel Banister described her personal experiences in devastating terms – in the British Medical Journal in 2021 – when she tried to gain help for her daughter, who had an eating disorder.[92] She wrote of the 'torments of mental illness within what is arguably, a chaotic, severely underfunded and too often barbaric system of mental health care.' She eventually gained help from the Royal Free Hospital Eating Disorder Service, but only after several frustrating months.

Repeated government promises of 'parity of esteem' between physical and mental illness services have a long way to go. The CQC report of 2022/23 writes of inpatient care where 'the quality of care is often not good enough.' Safety continues to be an area of concern, with 40% of providers rated as 'requires improvement' or 'inadequate for safety.' Parity of esteem is of *such significance*, yet it is so far from reality that the time is long overdue for improvements.

Proposals for Change

There is a clear, cost-effective gain to be made by investing in the most effective treatment and cure for anxiety and depression, namely Talking Therapies or Cognitive Behaviour Therapy (CBT).[93, 94] Increasing the number of clinical psychologists who lead this work will achieve this. It would seem to be a no-brainer were it not for the fact that savings to the exchequer from those returning to work will have to be made at the expense of the Department of Health. Joined-up thinking across departments is what is required. We will see whether a future government's promises to correct this problem will be fulfilled.

Meanwhile, the current situation should not be allowed to continue. The rapid release from mental hospitals of people with autism and learning difficulties should now be given the highest priority. Not only is it what they and their families deserve, it would release much-needed beds. Investment in regional speciality services for them and for those with eating disorders and personality disorders has been shown to be effective and is urgently needed more widely.

Making mental health nursing a more attractive career will be necessary if the service is to attract enough recruits. Currently, there are too many vacancies to ensure a safe and satisfying service. One way to encourage recruitment could be to introduce an accelerated progression through the grades of mental health nurses so that they reach higher levels and higher pay while remaining involved in clinical care. One hopes that this might be acceptable to the nursing profession.

Much is often made of prevention as a way of reducing ill health. Nowhere is this more true than in childhood, where mental disturbances too often lead to adult mental ill health. Investment in the early detection and treatment of disturbances in childhood and adolescence has been shown to have long-term benefits, and it is where investment now could bear dividends. 'The Incredible Years' experiment in which parents of children with severe behavioural disturbances were helped to manage their children reaped long-term benefits as the children matured. This scheme has fallen off the funding ladder but is of such potential benefit to society that it should now be revived.

Cardiff University is just one good example of how research using the long-term screening of all Welsh schoolchildren can uncover the causes of mental disturbances leading to their successful management. Early detection is the key, and more widespread adoption of screening techniques in schoolchildren and university students should lead to improved prevention of adult disease. Schools and universities may need help; they could do much more given additional support and resources.

There is much more to be done to ensure the parity of esteem between physical and mental illness; the lack of parity has long been seen as a serious defect. And even leaving aside the enormous value to individual patients by relieving their suffering, the return of very many to the productive workforce must be a huge inducement.

It will cost money, but the government should think of the return they will make on their investment.

Summary

I am far from the first to draw attention to the fact that we are failing to fulfil the idea of parity of esteem between mental and physical illness. Anxiety and depression are extremely common, yet too many patients wait far too long for treatment. Talking therapies are very effective, and at least 50% of patients return to productive work after a six-week course. Greater investment in clinical psychologists now would yield welcome dividends to the treasury.

Too many people with autism and ADHD are locked away unnecessarily in mental hospitals. It is widely regarded as a blot on society, and they should now be released to their families or cared for in the community.

Mental health nursing is not regarded as an attractive occupation, and urgent steps should be taken to correct this. Increasing retention and recruitment by improving conditions of service, the prospects of career progression, and relevant pay rewards should all be considered.

The mental health of children is a key determinant of health in later life. Greater effort is needed to detect mental disturbances in children in schools but will require the involvement and training of teachers in greater numbers. Attention now to the treatment of children and adolescents with drug addiction and anti-social behaviour can improve their life chances.

CHAPTER 6
MATERNITY SERVICES

Patient Experiences

As with mental health, maternity services have come in for criticism. The Care Quality Commission reported, in October 2023, that 10% of maternity units had an overall quality rating of 'inadequate', and that 39% 'require improvement'.[16] These figures included a 15% rating of 'inadequate' for safety of care; a rise from 4% in 2021. Only 3% of units were graded as 'outstanding' and 47% as 'good'. Poor quality of care was directly attributable to staff shortages.

A more recent study by CQC (February 2024) of patients' experiences of childbirth showed some improvements in the care received since the previous year.[95] However, they were still worse – overall – than five years ago, with many disturbing and persistent problems. For example, a quarter felt vulnerable when they were left alone after their childbirth.

Staff Under Pressure

Despite many staff working above and beyond the norm, the pressure from understaffing overwhelmed their capacity to provide safe and effective care. Midwives increasingly feel anxious and exhausted as they struggle to cover their clinical responsibilities with insufficient numbers. This is spelt out in stark detail in The All Party Parliamentary Group on 'Safe Staffing: The Impact of Staff Shortages on Maternity and Maternal Care'.[96] It is not a good way to provide high-quality care.

Impact of Deprivation and Race

The net result of their enquiry led CQC to express their concern about a continued decline in the experiences of women over the previous five years. Data from 2021 revealed a rise in stillbirth rates for the first time in seven years, and maternal deaths were rising too. This was particularly the case for areas with high deprivation rates; women in these areas were 2.5 times more likely to die than those in the least deprived areas. Black and Asian minorities were especially vulnerable. A report by MBRRACE, (Mothers and Babies: Reducing Risk through Audit and Confidential Enquiries) in October 2023 revealed the shocking data that black women were four times more likely to die during or after pregnancy than white women, while women of asian origin were twice as likely to die.[97] There is more than a hint that racial discrimination plays a role as black women feel that their concerns are ignored. It is not easy to understand these discrepancies when a high proportion of midwives, in London at least, are black.

Since 2012, the report noted there has been a continuing increase in the number of women dying from eclampsia, a treatable or preventable disease. Deaths associated with pre-eclampsia were four times greater in 2022 than in 2012.

Another major cause of death – that of suicide between six weeks and twelve months after the end of pregnancy – speaks for a failure of post-natal care.

Stillbirth and neonatal rates varied remarkably across the country, but babies of black ethnicity were more than twice as likely to be stillborn compared with white babies. Stillbirth rates are, unsurprisingly, highest in areas of deprivation. The safety of neonatal units is also under threat from understaffing. A third of neonatal nurses' shifts were understaffed.

Continuity of care for a pregnant woman by a named midwife is no longer the norm, and midwives have not been slow to point out that safety of care may be compromised.[96] A number of maternity units are threatened with closure because of inadequate staffing levels. The media have also not been slow in reporting the disastrous failures of maternity services in several centres around England, and the Ockenden Report on the failures in Nottingham is awaited with some trepidation. The debate in the House of Lords on maternity services on the 25th of January 2024 was sobering as some of the defects described above were spelt out.[98]

Overall, in maternity services, a lack of enough staff is associated with delays in care, poor communication, and a lack of one-to-one care from a named midwife. It is a sad tale of worry and concern within a vitally important workforce.[99]

The situation is exacerbated by the schism between obstetricians and midwives that has grown in recent years. Collaboration is under stress in too many maternity units, and a lack of leadership is damaging patient care.

Proposals for Change

Nowhere is the need for more staff and better motivated staff than in maternity care. A service with midwives who report high levels of stress, who are unhappy with the care they can provide, and concerned about their inadequate numbers, is bound to be one where complaints are far too common.

What is needed is not only more recruitment but a greater effort to retain staff. Pressures on existing staff can only be reduced when there are sufficient numbers of them and when their satisfaction levels improve so they are better motivated. A more enlightened approach to relieving the debt incurred by midwives during their training might encourage much-needed recruitment.

It is not as if recommendations have not been made. We have the 'Maternity Transformation Programme', a 'Long Term Plan', 'Better Birth', and a multi-year 'National Maternity Strategy' beginning in 2016 that has injected over £28 million of extra money into maternity care. The Times Health Commission's recommendation to offer relief for the payback of student fees for health care workers would help, too, and should be taken up by government.

But it is clear that there is much more that is still required. Attention has to be paid to reducing the racial discrimination that is such a blemish on the service. This, as with many other aspects of care, will rely on effective clinical leadership. This has to come especially from obstetricians and senior midwives, and the tendency for stand-offs between them should be urgently repaired. This falls to the leadership of the Royal College of Obstetricians and the Royal College of Nursing and Midwifery to press for change.

The commissioners of the service should be driving and monitoring this change. Safety concerns and poor communication should be high on those commissioners' agendas. But are the ICBs willing and able to bring the parties together?

Recent proposals to instigate a network of specialist centres with the aim of halving the unacceptable levels of maternal deaths are a reaction to deficiencies but will be a step in the right direction when it is put into action.[100] There is also the Government's 'NHS Long Term Workforce Plan' that envisages a marked increase in midwifery training places by 2031. That is a long time to wait for the urgent problems facing this service, and more action must be taken to improve working conditions that encourage and support existing staff so that they feel appreciated and more involved in decisions. This requires better leadership alongside support and monitoring by the commissioners.

Better maternal care has wide repercussions. Not only are mothers' experiences improved, but the future health of their babies is made much better, too. In utero health of the foetus determines future well-being of the child and, later, the adult. The adverse effects of drinking alcohol during pregnancy, clearly shown in 'foetal alcohol' syndrome, the neural tube defects in babies borne of mothers lacking folic acid, and the tragedy of the stunted limbs of babies borne of mothers given thalidomide, are obvious examples. Less obvious is the discovery that undernutrition during pregnancy may lead to increased incidences of hypertension, diabetes and heart disease in later life.[101] The 'Barker' hypothesis (David Barker) was based on evidence of this relationship, and although there is a little controversy surrounding the interpretation of his findings, they are sufficiently persuasive for preventive action to be taken during pregnancy.

Summary

The CQC assessments of maternity care reveal an unsatisfactory picture of variable and, too often, poor standards of care. There is evidence, too, of worse outcomes amongst black and other ethnic mothers.

Many of the problems can be ascribed to poor levels of staffing and low morale. Solutions will depend on making midwifery a more satisfying career. Attention to career prospects in the profession, to clinical leadership, and to repairing the damaging and perennial divisions between midwives and obstetricians. The Nursing and Midwifery Council and the Royal College of Obstetrics and Gynaecology should be tasked to examine how divisions can be repaired. The health of neonates clearly influences health in later life. It is vital that we give them the best start possible.

CHAPTER 7
PUBLIC HEALTH

Two obvious successes of Public Health have been government actions on smoking and the wearing of seat belts. But a less-than-perfect response to the outbreak of Covid in 2019 exposed glaring weaknesses.

The message that prevention is better than cure is very clear, even though it is hedged by difficulties in execution.

There are many determinants of health that are not susceptible to actions by Public Health bodies or the NHS. Poverty, educational attainment, unemployment, housing, and social class are probably more important. These determinants of health and mortality are spelt out in devastating detail by Michael Marmot in his books, 'Status Syndrome' and 'The Health Gap'. He emphasises the fact that messages that encourage better behaviour – in diet, exercise, and modes of living, for example – are unlikely to be sufficient to make the necessary changes. It depends *less* on the public's personal preferences in complying with messages put out by the Department of Health about how to live healthier lives and *more* on their circumstances, characterised by social deprivation, disadvantage, and powerlessness.

If we are to improve the health of the population at large, it will depend more on government actions than those of Public Health bodies.

Our seeming inability to curb burgeoning obesity rates in the UK is a case in point. Measures of rates of obesity reveal that it was much more frequent in 2023 than a year earlier. Between May and December 2022, there were many more deaths than the average over the previous five years. (Thirty-eight thousand excess deaths in the over 65s.) Some of the 13.5% increase recorded in December may have been due to a failure to account for the different age distribution of the populations at different times, but even when it is taken into account (using age-standardised mortality rates), it was still 5.8% higher.

These higher rates were not all accounted for by the Covid infection, and most were attributed to obesity-related diseases such as diabetes and heart attacks.

The incidence of death due to alcohol-related diseases, particularly cirrhosis of the liver, has gone up and down over the years. The incidence of alcohol consumption correlates very closely and inversely with the tax and cost of alcoholic drinks.[102] Whenever the Government has raised duty on alcohol, it has been followed by a fall in deaths due to liver disease. The argument in favour of raising duty in line with the cost of living is incontrovertible, but the Government of the day has often been reluctant to take on the drinks industry. It may not be entirely irrelevant that many in the media and politics enjoy a drink or two, as well! The health of the public suffers because of this inaction.

The problems are compounded by the attractiveness of eating, drinking alcohol and, for some, consuming drugs.

Public Health officials are struggling to get their healthy living messages across. They should, of course, continue to seek novel ways of providing information and persuade local authorities to offer swimming pools, gyms, and recreational facilities. But they should also continue to press government to take action. Government was successful in legislating against smoking, although there is still more to do there, but now they should press harder on factors that lead to high carbohydrate intake in children. Pressure on the industry to reduce the sugar content of soft drinks, cakes, and biscuits, the removal of 'tuck' shops and hamburger outlets near schools, and the provision of healthy foods in schools cannot be said to be entirely novel ideas, but they should now be more fully implemented. So much of adult ill health starts in unhealthy habits in childhood, and it is here where Public Health activity is focussing. So much of what is needed in the public health arena was spelt out in the far-seeing 'Acheson Report' of 1998.[103] It is well worth reading now.

Community-Acquired Infectious Diseases

So far as threats from infectious diseases are concerned, an uncertain grip on preventive measures against such outbreaks may have been taken since the Covid outbreak, but only belatedly. With yet another reorganisation of Public Health services, it remains to be seen whether such measures will be effective, and doubts are already being raised about our preparedness for a recrudescence of Covid.

The reasons why we were so inadequately prepared for Covid in 2019 are dealt with later, but the impact was devastating. The number of deaths from Covid was in the order of 230,600 by mid-November 2023 as confused and conflicting messages emanated from government and their advisors. Lockdowns and messages about isolation were late and oscillated between on and off. Nursing and care home occupants were particularly badly affected as infection spread rapidly through them, and many deaths followed.

The inadequate supply of protective clothing for staff left many feeling very vulnerable, and infection rates and deaths in staff were high. The net result was the loss of staff due to sickness and the inevitable increase in pressure on remaining staff.

By the time the successful vaccination programme was underway, Britain was thought to be one of the worst-performing countries in Europe in terms of its lack of preparedness and high death rates, although recent re-assessments suggest that Britain did not lag behind other European countries.

It is, however, increasingly clear that the UK was grossly ill-prepared for the outbreak of Covid. It took far too long to decide to extend testing for the public at large, but even then, it was the availability of tests and laboratories to carry them out that were soon shown to be inadequate. There were many other deficiencies that came to light, including a lack of beds, especially intensive care beds. Even at the time, there were warnings that the way the Government was dealing with the crisis was inadequate.[104, 105]

That the Government was very late in its response is clear; the scientific advice on which it relied was not always free of errors.

What had been lauded as the UK's pre-eminence in preparedness for pandemics was shown to be sadly lacking. Part of the problem was a lack of clear leadership and the multiplicity of bodies with different responsibilities. Public Health England might have been thought of as the natural lead body, but its role was of minor significance. It was barely visible in the myriad of bodies with responsibilities for dealing with the epidemic. Indeed, an incomprehensible number of agencies were involved. While it was responsible for developing tests for the virus and authorising laboratories to carry them out, Public Health England had no practical role in carrying out the tests. That was handed to 'Track and Trace', while procuring protective equipment lay separately under the purview of the Department of Health and Social Care. Co-ordination between these bodies was far from slick.

That is the bare outline of a highly complicated set of organisations, committees, advisors, and advisory boards that were involved in one way or another.

Protection of the public against infectious diseases had been eroded over many years. The Covid pandemic simply exposed its defects.

Public Health Laboratory Service

A Public Health Laboratory was set up in 1940 in response to the threat of bacterial warfare. With the start of the NHS in 1948, the Public Health Laboratory Service (PHLS) was established with its nerve centre laboratory in Colindale, North London.[106] It developed a remarkable reputation by combining, in the same buildings, its laboratory of leading microbiologists with a centre of excellence in epidemiology. It relied heavily on its own network of laboratories – based widely and strategically in every part of the country – and because of them, it was able to detect outbreaks of common and rare infections wherever they occurred anywhere in the land. They had all the expertise to detect outbreaks of infections, such as E. coli and Campylobacter, to monitor food and water supplies, and to provide vaccination programmes and protective advice. They were ideally placed to track and trace outbreaks.

The central reference laboratory was able to carry out all the highly specialised sub-typing of the samples sent to it from its laboratory network so that an accurate picture could be gained for the epidemiologists to trace the spread, and point to the source of infections rapidly. It became the envy of the world; even the Centre for Disease Control (CDC) in Atlanta, America, admired our combination of a central reference laboratory linked to what they lacked – the national network of Public Health laboratories.

It evolved in that format until 2003, when it was drastically revised and morphed into the Health Protection Agency (HPA). Some changes were valuable. The inclusion of protection against radiation and chemical hazards widened its responsibilities and made sensible use of the existing expertise in epidemiology. However, the pruning of the national network of Public Health laboratories on which the PHLS had relied was extremely damaging. The 31 district laboratories dedicated to public health surveillance were abolished, and their roles transferred to routine hospital laboratories. The eight regional laboratories were saved, but deprived of the support of local input, they were left to flounder. The functions of the PHLS network were all to be undertaken by routine laboratory staff based in hospitals. The latter, however, lacked the specific expertise required and failed to think of these public health functions as important. The commissioners and funders of care had responsibilities for a public health dimension in their hospital contracts, but it soon became obvious that they were distracted by the need to focus on direct patient care when funding was constrained.

The roles and responsibilities to track and trace that had been lost were just those that would have been invaluable in dealing with the Covid epidemic. But, in 2004, the Chief Medical Officer of the time advised government that we no longer needed the network and that routine hospital laboratories could cope. How misjudged that turned out to be! The decision has reverberated down the years, and the damage it caused has been starkly exposed by the Covid outbreak. If I appear bitter here, I should reveal a bias; I was Chair of the Board of the PHLS at the time and resigned in protest.

That was not to be the end of revisions to the organisation. Ten years later, the HPA was changed into Public Health England (PHE), which was split up so that part of it moved under local authorities' responsibility. Directors of Public Health were no longer employed by the NHS but by local authorities. Little wonder then that public health would suffer as government funding for local authorities was cut by 25% over the following ten years. This combination of inadequate funding, together with a loss of distributed expertise in a network of laboratories, placed the UK in a poor position to deal with emerging microbial threats. In a panic, after the debacle following Covid in 2021, PHE was disbanded and its roles subsumed into two new bodies, the more forward-sounding National Institute for Health Protection, subsequently renamed the UK Health Security Agency (UKHSA), and the Office for Health Promotion, subsequently renamed the Office for Health Improvement and Disparities (OHID). You could not make this up, and it does suggest a degree of panic in government circles. That over half a million pounds was spent on advice from McKinsey for the changes underlined government uncertainty. It remains to be seen whether these organisations will live up to their names and prove effective or, indeed, whether they will survive.

Experience suggests that changing the names of health organisations is rarely productive and is almost always disruptive as staff become confused about their responsibilities as they are released and re-employed. And the service is hardly ever improved. There are too many examples, as I elucidate later, where repeated re-organisations have created expensive disruption with little or no perceptible gain.

I suggest now some ideas about how we can begin to regain the trust and reliance we desperately need in our public health protection services.

Proposals for Change

It was in recognition of the breadth of the responsibilities of Public Health England that led to it being divided into two distinct entities, and we should examine whether both of the roles they play should continue to remain within local authorities.

The responsibilities of the Health Security Agency require expertise in microbiology, epidemiology, and chemical and radiological hazards. Currently, it depends on microbiologists in NHS hospitals for the detection of infectious disease outbreaks. That this was inadequate was clearly demonstrated in the near absence of 'track and trace' of patients during the onset of Covid when co-ordination between PHE and the NHS was poor. There is a clear need now to set up microbiological laboratory functions that are specifically designed to detect outbreaks of infections, for example, from contaminated food and water supplies, and to pick up rare or previously unknown infections. The

Central Reference Laboratory in Colindale, North London, is rightly world-renowned for its highly specialised microbiological testing linked to epidemiological expertise. But they are entirely dependent on a network of facilities around the country to detect outbreaks and the breakdown of that network has limited the capacity of the Central Reference Laboratory to do its work. Replacing the network now would go a long way to ensuring that the protection of the public against future outbreaks would become a reality. Since microbiology training is an NHS responsibility, it makes sense to bring the Health Security Agency within the NHS. The new laboratory function could be housed within existing hospitals, and new buildings may not be needed. But their funding and functions would have to be ring-fenced. Within the NHS, they would not have to compete for the more severely stretched resources of the local authority.

Public Health Board Remits

The 'OHI and D' has a much wider remit than detecting outbreaks of infectious diseases and depends not only on public health professionals but general practitioners and other departments of state. Discrepancies in mortality rates between deprived and affluent parts of the country exemplify the fact that many non-clinical factors contribute to the well-being of society, including poverty, deprivation, poor housing, racism, and unemployment.

GPs, health visitors and district nurses are on the front line in detecting preventable causes of disease. It is they who, if not distracted and overloaded, can detect and advise heavy smokers and those with obesity and alcoholism. The 'Quality and Outcomes Framework' is supposed to incentivise GPs for this public health function.

The difficult job of trying to change the behaviour of the public at large falls on 'OHI and D'.

It is not as if people are unaware of the dangers of overeating junk foods, excess alcohol consumption, or the need for exercise. It is getting the message across sufficiently strongly that is so difficult. It is, however, where the most focus should be directed, and recourse to commercial advertising agencies whose job it is to influence behaviour could be fruitful. But it is from the influence that the public health community can have on government that more radical improvements can come. Action on poor housing, better local transport, and limitations on industry in their production of foods heavy in sugar and salt can bear dividends.

Proposals to increase the sugar tax and to press industry to reduce the calorie content of soft drinks is a government responsibility, as is pressure to reduce the availability of junk food outlets near schools. They should now fully accept this responsibility and act.

The use of individualised e-messages to vulnerable populations has a role and should now be activated. It is particularly important to aim public health messages at schoolchildren and their parents. Greater effort should be made to instil healthy living practices in youngsters, where they are likely to have the most impact in later life. Keeping teachers well-informed with health messages is vital. Training sessions for staff with regular updates could help.

Immunisation and Screening

Falling rates of immunisation in childhood have followed false claims of potential dangers, particularly the MMR vaccination. Greater effort to refute such claims will require a much stronger PR campaign. At the moment, the battle is being lost on the internet as negative propaganda dominates. Rising rates of measles infections are worrying. A renewed effort to spread positive messages will require novel approaches to try to influence public opinion. Public Health staff are entirely knowledgeable and capable but must now be given the tools and support they need to innovate with messaging to the public and specific subgroups at risk.

Not all health screening techniques are necessarily valuable. Proponents of breast screening for every woman and PSA screening for all men for prostate cancer have been challenged to demonstrate the evidence that they save lives. But screening for specific subsets of the vulnerable population is where effort should be focussed. It would save money as well as avoid the unnecessary worry inflicted on healthy individuals. However, the widespread use of tests of stools for occult blood (FIT) does pick up a proportion of patients with bowel cancer and should be publicised more widely.

In the elderly, screening for osteoporosis can bear dividends in the prevention of fractures. It is limited by the availability of bone scanners, and their numbers should be boosted. There are just too few of them at present.

Programmes promoting increased exercise and activity should be spread more widely, and the early detection of falls with simple home monitors should be boosted.[107] This is where Public Health staff are in a good position to draw attention to these simple measures. They are also able to bring poor and unhealthy housing to the attention of local authorities. They should be given greater powers to intervene where they find the health of residents is threatened. But it will be important, too, to ensure that 'wokeism' does not interfere with good practice. An example occurred when a social worker proposed tagging a dementia sufferer so that her family could keep track of her as she wandered off on her own. The local council vetoed it on the grounds that this interfered with her personal freedom.

Public Health doctors and their staff are often starved of funds as they try to fulfil their wide responsibilities. Cash-strapped local authorities should strongly consider the idea of ring-fenced funding for this vital role that they play, as much as ring-fencing may be disliked.

Summary

There can be few people who are unaware that smoking, drinking alcohol, and eating too much high-calorie food can damage their health. So, simply putting out more advice on healthy living is of only limited value. It required government action – over decades – to have a positive impact on smoking habits, and it will probably need government action to boost healthy living, for example, to put pressure on industry to reduce the sugar content of soft drinks and to limit the presence of fast food outlets near schools. Alcohol consumption falls as duty on it rises. Increasing duty reduces the incidence of cirrhosis in later years and government should abandon their reluctance to raise duty in line with inflation.

The response to the Covid outbreak was suboptimal. Efforts should now be made to re-instate a network of Public Health laboratories across the country to monitor food and water supplies, and to track and trace outbreaks of common and rare infectious diseases. The *lack* of such facilities contributed to the poor response to the Covid outbreak.

Greater efforts are needed to counteract the negative propaganda levelled against vaccination and immunisation. Contemporary methods of transmitting messages using social media may be valuable.

Amongst their many important roles, health visitors are on the front line in drawing attention to problems that lead to ill health, including poor housing and unsanitary living conditions. It is unhelpful that their numbers have been falling and further attention should be given to increasing their numbers.

CHAPTER 8
TRUST AND MISTRUST

One of the most serious consequences of the deterioration in staff relations is the increasing mistrust that permeates the service. It is not only the distrust of government by doctors and nurses, or the demeaning opinion of the doctors by ministers and civil servants, it is also inter-professional mistrust that sometimes undermines essential collaboration in patient care.

Patients' Reliance on Trust

When patients rely on the close collaboration between caring professionals, any sense of mistrust is very unnerving.

Nurses are not always sympathetic towards doctors, whom they may see as aloof and superior, while doctors sometimes seem to regard nurses as uncooperative or unavailable. Not everywhere – and not every doctor or nurse, of course – and it may be thought that I exaggerate to make the case. But it is undoubtedly true that there is a simmering undercurrent of suspicion between the two. The mistrust between midwives and obstetricians is too damaging to be allowed to continue.

Less doubtful is the far too common antipathy between the 'managers' and the medical staff. Both are stressed, and communication between them often becomes impersonal and bureaucratic. Commands from on high do not go down well. Nor do the actions of recalcitrant doctors gain any favours. Misunderstandings follow a lack of communication, so the system lurches on in frustration on both sides.

But the deepest mistrust is evident in the ways in which governments and their ministers are held by doctors and nurses. Ministers and their civil servants do not seem to have much time for the medical and nursing professions and, hence, can easily ignore them. The BMA is seen purely as a trade union, entirely responsible for the salaries and well-being of its members, while the medical Royal Colleges are viewed as bastions of privilege. That doctors can be awkward at times is hardly doubted. As highly educated, individualistic professionals, they can easily be seen as intransigent, but that does not excuse governments from ignoring them.

Announcing Health Bills with little or no consultation is certain to be received with antipathy, but it is most often due to the reluctance to accept untested reforms delivered from on high that leads to mistrust. To the medical profession, it often seems that their concerns are cursorily dismissed. That is not a good way to encourage collaboration. Resistance to untested reform is common and mostly justified. In contrast, most innovations in patient care arise from the inspiration of doctors and nurses and their use of research evidence rather than from Acts of Parliament. Almost any advance in care that can be mentioned does not come from government initiatives. Dramatic advances in childhood leukaemia, in breast and other cancers, in angiography and angioplasty, in minimally invasive surgery, scanning, and fibreoptics have all arisen from research and adoption into clinical practice. And there are many more.

A lack of trust manifests in many ways, mostly to the detriment of patients and their care.

Doctors and nurses do not always behave well, and trust is easily lost. We have had several high-profile cases of gross misconduct in recent years. Dr. Harold Shipman, convicted in January 2000, and Lucy Letby very recently, were murderers who took too long to be discovered. The inquiry after the Shipman case resulted in a dramatic shakeup of the doctors' regulatory body, the GMC. This was on the very uncertain presumption that doctors intent on murder would be deterred by a 'strengthened' GMC. Much expensive browbeating to satisfy the public, but to doubtful impact on doctors intent on murder.

There are very many more examples of less serious demeanours in which patients have suffered because of mistakes, errors of judgement, or malice. Many of these come up before the medical insurance organisations, the Medical Protection Society, the Medical Defence Union, and the General Medical Council. Although simple human error may lie behind many of these cases and although the number of such cases seems large, especially in their reporting in the media, it is the case that compared with the total number of doctor- or nurse-patient interactions, the denominator – the fraction of those causing harm – is very small.

Responses to Poor Behaviour

Sadly, nowhere has it been possible to retain a sense of perspective in the response to well-publicised transgressions (no matter how rare they are). The response to a single and possibly unique event in which a Liverpool pathologist retained pathology specimens from children in the boot of his car was not only to set up an inquiry into how it had happened, entirely appropriately, but then the Government saw fit to produce a new Act of Parliament. 'The Human Tissues Act' was to take a huge mallet to crack a significant but minute nut.

There have been no similar cases since then, but nor had there been any before that. The Act did, however, cause considerable distraction for many in pathology departments across the country as they were forced to examine their stores of pathology specimens and offer them back to patients or their next of kin. Patients can be forgiven for being surprised to be offered their biopsies, surgical specimens, and moles. A completely new and distracting bureaucracy has arisen as a result. Expensive and time-consuming, it has done little to improve the safety or management of the service.

Bureaucracy has always been an issue in the NHS and the BMJ reported, in 2010, that a list of no less than 30 regulators, auditors, inspectorates and accreditation agencies were about to be abolished.[108]

Many of these bodies requested the same information that was then squirrelled away, never to be looked at again. Some of them have disappeared, but others have sprung up in their place. 'Bonfires' of quangos always seem to be on the agenda.[109] It is hard to escape the conclusion that no one in the NHS is to be trusted and an expensive and distracting industry has been set up to keep check on everyone and everything. If ever there is money to be saved, look no further.

It seems that all governments are experts at dreaming up bright ideas – the world is full of those with bright ideas –

but what they singularly lack is a clear understanding of how to implement them.

Improving Trust

Implementation is entirely dependent on winning the hearts and minds of those who are expected to do the implementing; in this case, it is those at the coal face: the nurses, doctors, and other health professionals. When ministers no longer have much trust in the professions, as sometimes seems to be the case, then it is little wonder that bright ideas fail to be implemented. Businesses that are successful know full well that they must take their staff with them. It is also the case that in other industries where emotional stress levels are high, planning of the workforce often includes a 20% numerical uplift. The NHS and social care exemplify workforces that are under emotional stress. This is a concept that sadly eludes many health ministers. Later, I outline some possible ways in which we might mitigate these problems for the NHS.

Summary

Regaining trust once it has been lost is extraordinarily difficult. Yet patients rely on the trust they have in those who care for them and that, in turn, is dependent on the perception they have of the *trust that exists between their carers*.

The causes of mistrust within medicine are multiple, as described in this chapter. Mistrust between government and the caring professions will only be assuaged with evidence of improved collaboration and more inspiring leadership on both sides. It will take time. Similarly, an improvement in trust between nurses and doctors will only follow improved leadership, more opportunities for closer working in teams, and opportunities for regular formal and informal discussions. Meetings for that to occur should be instituted.

Mistrust, wherever it occurs in health and social care, can only damage patient care.

CHAPTER 9
MEDICAL RESEARCH

Markers of Excellence

Advances in treatment and cures in the NHS depend heavily on research, and – on the face of it – Britain is very well placed to undertake much of it. We have a large population of patients in the NHS, most of whom are ready and willing to engage in the research effort and who are theoretically happy to volunteer for clinical trials. There are several invaluable funding streams accessible, too. The Association of Medical Research Charities represents over 100 medical charities, including such mega-charities as the Wellcome Trust, British Heart Foundation, and Cancer Research UK; together they fund £1.55 billion of research per annum.

Clearly, charities are keen to support research into the diseases they collect funds for. Government funding is significant, too. The National Institute for Health and Care Research provides £1.324 billion, and the Medical Research Council £599 million per annum. These sources are in addition to the pharmaceutical industry's investment in research and development in the UK, which amounted to some £5 billion in 2020. On every measure of research output and success, the UK is high on the list of countries active in research.

But despite all these positive virtues, the UK fails to achieve its full potential. It could do so much better since many of its problems are soluble.

Clinical Commitments Dominate

Even without the impact of medical staff strikes during 2023/24, the excessive load of patient care under which most operate has made it extremely difficult, if not impossible, for clinicians, and not only doctors, to engage in research. Even when interest is ignited, clinical workloads are heavy and distracting.

For trainees, the situation is compounded by the rigidity and formality of their training programmes. Subjected to multiple rotations to gain a range of experiences, often in a variety of hospitals and institutions, any thoughts of research have to be abandoned. Postgraduate Deans, who are responsible for ensuring that the training programmes fulfil all the requirements of the GMC and Royal Colleges, stick to their formulae. The flexibility needed to fit research in is not readily found. Little wonder I am told that the major funding bodies, including the Medical Research Council and the Wellcome Trust, have curtailed their funding for clinical research fellowships. They see little value in investing in these types of fellowships when the pressures on clinicians to complete their training and care for patients are so distracting.

The Times Health Commission recommends that doctors be given up to 20% of their time to engage in research. An invaluable proposal, but one that is unlikely to be achievable within available resources.

Clinical research is seen as the province of those in academic posts – lectureships and the like – but they also often carry a heavy clinical load that limits their capacity to conduct research. Only in relatively large academic departments is it possible, for example, to rotate fellows through clinical and research responsibilities.

Bureaucracy

The effort required to gain the approval of research ethics committees is daunting. The committees themselves have been streamlined in their approach, but the mountains of forms to be completed are time-consuming beyond what anyone but a dedicated bureaucrat would find reasonable or proportionate. The Research and Innovation Committees set up in University Hospitals have done little to reduce the paperwork. Ostensibly there to help support researchers, they require multiple forms to be completed, too, before approval can be given. They are creatures of the NHS rather than the Universities, and it is likely that their intention is to ensure that any clinical research does not consume NHS resources.

Research in Primary Care

Research in general practice is similarly threatened. It is only the unusual GP who has been able to take on a research role. There are some very good examples of academic departments of general practice engaged in high-quality and important research, but outside academe, it is much less obvious. They receive little recognition, training or recompense for so doing. This is not a recent phenomenon, of course. It is hardly surprising that very few have enrolled their patients in clinical trials despite the advantages of engaging the potentially huge number of patients for whom they care.

It is the sad case, too, that GPs have historically been bastions of resistance to using their patient data for research. Their defence has always been that they must act as the guardians of their patients' confidentiality. Despite numerous efforts, including Acts of Parliament, Data Guardians, Caldicott regulations and the like, that resistance has been barely overcome (except in Scotland). Much invaluable research, involving clinical trials, disease epidemiology, and new treatment evaluation, has been inhibited.

The exception to the general decline in capacity for clinical research occurred during the Covid epidemic. It was then that well-run clinical trials clearly demonstrated the value of corticosteroid drugs and novel nursing techniques in improving outcomes. They also showed that other drugs were *unhelpful*.

Clinical Trials and the Pharmaceutical Industry

Our inability to conduct large-scale clinical trials of new drugs is reflected in the increasing resistance of the pharmaceutical industry to invest in the UK. It has been estimated that the number of patients in clinical trials in the UK has fallen from 50,000 in 2018 to 28,000 in 2022.[110] The industry can find much more encouragement in other countries, and that is where they have moved their attention.

The attitude they meet in the NHS is not helped by the lingering suspicion amongst some in government, the public, and the medical profession, that industry is focussed too heavily on the profit motive. That data derived from patients will be used for commercial gain is seen as a danger and has bedevilled collaboration with industry. This suspicion may be reducing but still provides some background noise at a time when close working relations between industry, academe, and the NHS could be potentially very productive for new treatments and cures. Lord O'Shaughnessy's report provides a clear set of recommendations for government and others and should now be put into action.[110]

Biobank

That it is possible to gain consent for research from patients, including the future use of clinical data, was shown when 500,000 of the public agreed to engage with 'Biobank'. This organisation gained full consent to record the clinical history, lifestyle characteristics, and genetic information of all these volunteers. Again, there is a major impediment to Biobank gaining a full picture of patients' history. It lies in the resistance of GPs to allow access to the data they hold, even though their patients have given consent. The database, which in any case only includes de-identified details, is available for bona fide researchers and is a valuable resource for epidemiological studies, but it is incomplete because of the reluctance of GPs. It could be so much more valuable!

Biobank has received some 4,500 carefully vetted applications for research since it opened to researchers in 2012. Several thousand research papers have been produced on a variety of major topics, including cardiovascular disease, stroke, diabetes, and cancer. It is just this sort of consent from patients for the use of their data, suitably anonymised, that could make a difference to future research. It is regulatory bodies and some GPs who have placed limitations on access that are the bottleneck, and it will be of interest to see whether recent government offers of incentives to GPs to engage in clinical trials will prove effective.

Attracting Overseas Clinical Researchers

There is one other area of concern for clinical research in the UK.

Before Britain left the EU, doctors, including clinical researchers, could enter the UK to practise if they had completed the requisite number of years in their training and could pass an English language test. Now, they must join academic clinicians from the USA, Australia, and the rest of the world who go through the more rigid assessments required by the GMC.

The inflexibility of the system that has been set up has made it difficult for a distinguished professor in psychiatry, say, to come to Britain to engage in a collaborative research programme in dementia. The requirement that these highly-qualified clinical researchers must take further clinical training and examinations has proved too high a barrier for many when they consider whether to come to Britain. Collaborative research is thus prohibited by a rigid bureaucratic system that throttles cooperation and partnerships.

It is remarkable that, despite all the barriers I have described, so much excellent clinical research is performed in Britain. It is just that so much more could be achieved if we could overcome them.

Each of the problems I have outlined is potentially soluble.

But they do require action and not only by government. The medical profession, particularly the Medical Royal Colleges, the British Medical Association, the Postgraduate

Deans and the General Medical Council, as well as funding bodies, need to consider how they can help overcome these difficulties urgently. There are many valuable suggestions in the O'Shaughnessy Report[110] and The Academy of Medical Sciences paper.[111]

Proposals for Change and Summary

Medical research in the UK has much to be proud of. International comparisons reveal that it produces more advances in science than most similar Western countries. Yet, it could do much better if some of the constraints on it were overcome.

Research by clinicians is severely limited by the pressure to provide clinical care. Trainee doctors are also constrained by rigid training programmes. The Times Health Commission recommended that 20% of clinicians' time should be devoted to research. It is difficult to imagine where that 20% might come from, given the failure to provide enough care to meet the clinical demand.

Some relief for researchers could be obtained by reducing the bureaucratic hurdles that have to be overcome in gaining permission. Similarly, encouragement for GPs to allow the use of data derived from their patients for research is vital for clinical trials to be performed. Government inducements and reassurances about the safety and confidentiality of the use of patient data will be necessary. The GMC should pay attention to a more flexible approach to encourage senior overseas clinical researchers to come to work in the UK.

CHAPTER 10
RE-ORGANISATION AND RE-RE-ORGANISATION OF THE NHS

While my focus in this book is on patients and the staff caring for them, it is not possible to ignore the role of governments in their efforts to improve the service. That these have not always been successful is obvious from the number of times each new health secretary has felt the need to revise the system introduced by their predecessor.[112]

We have been through a 30-year period of the 'internal market' and 'purchaser-provider' split that has been so damaging, and we are only just emerging from it. It was all driven by a desire to 'make ends meet' under the limited resources made available.

Nick Timmins provides a clear and helpful description of the history of the Health Service since its inception in 1948. He interviewed a series of past health ministers and revealed how almost impossible their task is.[112] On the one hand, they are responsible to the taxpayer for a huge amount of public expenditure; at the same time, they have tried to devolve responsibility for delivering the service to the local level. Delegation downward and accountability upwards has never worked well, and ministers have always had to answer to Parliament for any failings. Policy and implementation have not always meshed, and health ministers have had the unenviable task of trying to make them work better.

Demand has always been expanding as the population ages, and the march of science has brought more and more expensive tests and treatments so that medical inflation has outpaced the inflation of other goods and services. Providing a service – free at the point of delivery – is always going to be a challenge, especially when governments have been reluctant to inflict higher taxes on a resistant public. Indeed, almost as soon as the euphoria of the new NHS in 1948 had settled, it was realised that it was unaffordable! Within a very short time, charges were introduced for prescriptions and dental and ophthalmic services.

A service described as 'administered' and delivered through Regional Hospital Boards lacked any sort of financial control. In an effort to introduce a 'managed' system, the 1974 reforms set up regional, area, and district health authorities. It seemed to be a simple and rational way of distributing resources based on a formula that included population numbers and indicators of deprivation. It soon became both politicised and overly bureaucratic. There was no real competition for funds amongst hospitals, and they did what they could with what they were given. A lack of control on spending became obvious, and the large teaching hospitals complained that they were not adequately recompensed for the extra work that was thrust upon them for specialised care from other districts.

Meanwhile, primary care and NHS community care were funded separately through their individual GP and Community Trust contracts, while social care was funded via local authorities. No one was entirely satisfied, and the Conservative Government of the 1980s – stepping in to try to introduce some market efficiencies – sought the help of Roy Griffiths, a senior manager at Sainsbury's supermarket. The Griffiths Report sharply pointed out the lack of any financial control, and it was this that opened the door to ideas of an internal market.

No thought seems to have been given as to how a market can work when neither the price to be charged nor the demand were under the control of anyone engaged in providing the service. The price was set centrally by the tariff for each item of care and the demand came from the public at the door. There was no one at the entrance to Emergency Departments controlling access. Rationing by the availability of resources (translated into waiting lists) was the only way control was exerted.

But the fuse was lit when Alain Enthoven's internal market idea was taken up enthusiastically by Prime Minister Margaret Thatcher, the grocer's daughter. Her health minister, Kenneth Clarke, put it into effect, and the basic principle has been sustained through a series of Acts of Parliament. Few, if anyone, took note of Tony Judt when he wrote that 'Markets do not automatically generate trust, co-operation or collective action for the common good.'[113]

Each of the ten or more bills introduced since then has involved a re-organisation of the structure of the NHS, each followed by a re-re-organisation (or re-disorganisation as Ray Tallis would have it) as each preceding system was found wanting in one way or another. Layers of administration were repeatedly formed and then disbanded with bewildering frequency, each lasting but three or four years. Each involved the expensive business of retirement and re-hiring of senior administrative staff as the names, and occasionally the function, of each layer of bureaucracy was altered.

No one paid much attention to what John Maynard Keynes had written, 'It is not sufficient that the state of affairs which we need to promote should be better than that which preceded it, it must be sufficiently better to make up for the evils of transition.' The evils of transition were felt at each turn of the screw that inhibited continuity of care. Local planning initiatives suffered, too. No minister in either of the main parties has been able to resist the pressure to inflict change on taking up office. Primary care has had fundholding GPs, Practice-Based Commissioning , Clinical Commissioning Groups and overarching Primary Care Trusts in which GPs have been asked to take charge of purchasing care for their patients. That they have been found wanting is clear from the number of iterations there have been. The number of bodies has expanded and contracted over the years.

It was Labour's Alan Milburn who stirred the pot further when he introduced 350 new Primary Care Trusts to replace 100 Health Authorities, set up 29 Strategic Health Authorities in place of eight Regional Bodies, and put up four new Regional Directorates. The turmoil introduced by these changes was resolved a couple of years later when these bodies were disbanded and a more limited number introduced. He had lost his way in a morass of conflicting advice and ideology.

But it was the Lansley reforms of 2012 that left a bigger mark. Andrew Lansley had taken a long-term interest in health services and was very well informed, albeit, as it turned out, misguided about what was needed. He set about removing several layers of bureaucracy that had accumulated over the years. Primary Care Trusts, Strategic Health Authorities, Regional Offices and NHS England were all abolished. It certainly saved money but also saw the loss of many highly-qualified managers following the inevitable purge. They were sorely missed in the gap as the new organisation was installed. The NHS Board took over, supposedly at arms' length from government, and at the other end, the new powerful GP Commissioning Groups were given responsibility for spending 80% of NHS funds; the remaining 20% was retained centrally to be spent on specialised services. The fact that the majority of GPs were independent contractors and not employed by the NHS did not dissuade Lansley from giving them responsibility for such a large proportion of NHS cash. Nor was the fact that most were inexperienced (and a few incompetent) a deterrent either.

Area Teams were invented to try to assist GPs, but it was how they should use all the cash available to them that caused so much dismay amongst many in the service. Lansley opened access further for private organisations to provide services. Competition was wide open for anyone with the relevant qualifications to bid for a service, and the newly introduced 'Monitor' was given responsibility for promoting such competition. The mandatory tendering process that followed was soon shown to be expensive and disruptive. Hospital trusts had to hire personnel and legal assistance to undertake the whole process of responding to tenders, all requiring resources. It was not as though there was no warning about the expense of commissioning. The Commons Select Committee Reports of 2010 and 2011 had said as much.[114, 115]

And hospital trusts faced the prospect of their services becoming disrupted as some elements were hived off to private providers. For example, a hospital losing some of its surgical specialties to a private provider would be hard to sustain. Income from private providers was to be limited to 49% of the total, but this cherry-picking inevitably distorted the range of services a hospital could provide. It is hard to imagine anything further from integration of services than mandatory tendering, and it was soon seen to be a damaging diversion.

Since then, the Government has been rowing back from the Lansley reforms. As the CCGs were revealed to lack sufficient expertise, they were slowly reduced in number and renamed as Sustainability and Transformation Partnerships before becoming Integrated Care Organisations. Integration was on the move, and while money might have been saved as management tiers were rationalised, some unmet needs were being revealed, taking up any savings.

Changes were also occurring in a number of local initiatives, so-called 'place-based initiatives', in a variety of efforts to integrate services. One of the most successful was developed in Salford, where Sir David Dalton, Chief Executive of Salford Royal Hospitals, with other leaders in the city successfully integrated NHS hospital and community services, including elements of general practice and social care.

These types of initiatives paved the way for the White Paper of February 2021, 'Integration and Innovation', and the Health and Care Bill that was widely welcomed later the same year. The net result was to see the management of the NHS come full circle from the internal market and back to one closely resembling the 1974 system of a regional tier associated with area health authorities. Not exactly the same, but near enough with ten regional offices instead of the original 14 Regional Health Authorities plus 42 Integrated Care Systems and their boards, in place of the Area or District Health Authorities of the 1970s. In truth, the need for a regional tier had never entirely disappeared and it persisted in various guises, including the earlier Regional Offices, the Strategic Health Authorities after 2001, and the Regional Teams, post-Lansley.

The changes saw the demise of a number of bodies concerned with managing the commercial aspects of the market. 'NHS Improvement', formed from a merger of Monitor and CQC, was simply taken into NHS England and the NHS Trust Development Authority disappeared. As the market was disassembled, the Competition and Markets Authority no longer had any role in monitoring such matters as mergers in the NHS.

Integrating care does not mean that the problems for patients and staff have been resolved. Nor does it mean that the conundrum of how to fund such an expensive service from extremely limited resources has been settled. It does mean, however, that the profligate 30-year experiment, with a range of models of an internal market, is no longer wasting money on its administration. As Calum Paton writes, 'It would have been more straightforward to develop 'integration' from (the pre-1990 system) as opposed to embarking on a tortuous 25-year tour of the variants of the market.'[116]

These damaging machinations also reveal another truth. What patients seek is a service that meets their needs and it is that, that should lead directly to the development of services to meet those needs. It should be followed by the management arrangements required to fulfil those aspirations, not *precede* them. In this light, concentrating first on the management arrangements is starting at the wrong end, yet this is what a succession of governments have been doing for far too long.

The recent Health Care Act, 2022, is a move in the right direction towards integration and away from market splits, but two obvious difficulties have not been covered. The first is the problem of how to repair the failures of recruitment and, in particular, the retention of staff. The second is the difficulty inherent in integrating the NHS with social care when the former is state-funded and the latter is means-tested. This is not helped by the way in which membership of the Integrated Care System is chosen. It includes a GP, a representative from the hospital trust, and one from a local authority. No one from Social Services – the provider of community care – is directly represented. A Director of Public Health acts in an advisory capacity but is not in a position to speak for the needs of the community sector. But until the NHS is fully integrated with social care, there will always be obstacles to the way both operate. They are interdependent and integration is essential in the long run. Furthermore, it has been shown to be achievable in at least one part of England and probably more.

As mentioned earlier, Salford Royal Hospitals, by this time already managing community health services, entered into a unique partnership with Salford City Council and the Salford Clinical Commissioning Group, which enabled the Salford Royal Trust to take over employer responsibility for all the social workers in the city. Bringing together the key elements of hospital, community health services, social care, and some parts of primary care meant that patient care was significantly streamlined. It enabled a single organisation to plan and deliver care to patients in a much more integrated way.

The majority of resources then sat in a single organisation, minimising tedious negotiations over funding between organisations. It began to bring staff together so that they worked in a single team. An innovative primary care practice was formed, with salaried GPs and other health care professionals, that enabled a focussed service to be provided to each nursing home and in support of care workers. And IT oiled the wheels as patient records were readily available across primary, community, and secondary care and into those in social care. All the city's pharmacies were also linked in, so that patients' drug records and whether they were taking up their prescriptions were accessible to their attendants.

Developments were also being pursued for integrated patient records, which – in part – enabled the internationally recognised Salford Lung Study, involving 80 GP practices and 130 pharmacies working together to pioneer a new approach to evaluating and improving the treatment of people with asthma and chronic obstructive pulmonary disease.

A number of factors contributed to this remarkable achievement.

Firstly, Dalton had been very successful in building good relationships with staff. He ensured that key medical, nursing, and other staff were all on board with him to improve standards of care. It took time. He was Chief Executive for 17 years during a period when most lasted barely three years in similar posts. It was this successful longevity, the co-operative teamworking in the Trust, and the interest in working in partnership with others in his locality that gave the local authority the confidence to transfer the management of social care.

It was not possible to avoid the financial constraints felt nationally, but there is little doubt that patient outcomes were improved and that staff satisfaction levels rose. It certainly prompted several visits by health ministers.

Salford was not the only place in England where a range of different approaches were being tried, but the question of how generalisable approaches might be – such as that developed in Salford – is more difficult to resolve. Years of mutual suspicion will be hard to overcome, and few local authorities would willingly give up responsibility for funds for social care to a hospital trust. And hospital trust managers would need to broaden their understanding of the differences in providing high standards of out-of-hospital care where the medical model is far less appropriate.

But pursuing new approaches to delivering truly integrated care must be the direction of travel. And it can be done, given excellent local leadership.

Summary

My only plea here is for the Government to avoid any suggestion of a further Bill to re-organise the NHS and social care.

Integration of the NHS and social and community care has always been highly desirable but never achievable. The new Integrated Care Boards are no doubt useful in encouraging joint working but do not have a great deal of influence on the behaviour of those at the coal face tasked with working together. My belief is that the only way successful integration might occur is by local initiatives.

That will depend on excellent and inspiring local leadership able to encourage hospital trusts and local authorities to pool their resources for the common good. It can be done, but it will require central government to ensure that the conditions for such local initiatives are promoted.

CHAPTER 11
FUNDING MATTERS

Many of this book's proposals for improving the care of patients and the welfare of staff do not require more money, but more funding is inevitably needed. That money does indeed talk was demonstrated when the Blair Government increased health spending to match European levels.[117] Patient satisfaction rose, waiting lists virtually disappeared, and GPs became accessible… until the funding faltered.

Here, I discuss where additional money might be found.

Pruning The Agencies

There has been more than one attempt to reduce the number of bodies concerned with supporting and regulating the NHS. At least two 'bonfires' of the agencies in the last few years were publicised only for others to accumulate in their wake.[118] It is difficult now to see where savings were made then, but with 25 agencies and bodies now supporting the work of the DHSC, it must be possible to seek savings by disbanding some of them.[119]

No doubt there will be resistance amongst those working in targeted organisations, but a clear-eyed examination of what roles they play and the impact (if any!) they have on the care or safety of patients must be a worthwhile exercise. An examination of their budgets suggests that savings made by abolishing all of them – something that may be impossible anyway – would save only millions of pounds; nowhere near enough to fund much of the shortfall in the NHS and social care budgets.

Litigation and 'No-Fault-Compensation'

NHS Resolution is responsible for settling negligence claims, amongst other roles. It paid out just under £2 billion in claims in 2022, but it has to make significant provision for future potential claims of almost £70 billion. The reasons for mounting negligence claims are not difficult to understand given the stresses and strains amongst staff in the NHS and care in the community. The budget of NHS Resolution is largely consumed by legal activities and it is here that criticisms have arisen.

In recent years, its funding has fluctuated (indeed, it is now lower than in some previous years), suggesting that there may be room for further stringencies. The recent suggestion to replace the current litigation process with a no-fault compensation system (that simply requires compensation without the admission of guilt and without the involvement of lawyers)[120] is an important proposal that is endorsed by The Times Health Commission. This must be the direction of travel for patients, staff, and health authorities if we are to relieve them of the tedious stress and cost of litigation. It has the potential to make considerable savings for the NHS. Other bodies concerned with negligence claims against clinicians – such as the Medical Protection Society or Medical Defence Union – take great care in assessing claims, and the role of the NHS Litigation Authority could be reduced if a no-fault scheme was introduced.

There are other bodies whose roles and responsibilities are worthy of a reassessment. I mention the Human Tissue Authority, whose budget is some £5.8 million per annum. It was set up as a knee-jerk reaction to a scandal in which an aforementioned Liverpool pathologist was found to have kept parts of the bodies of dead babies in the boot of his car. This scandal had not occurred before, nor has it done so since, but the Act has created a whole new regulatory edifice that has introduced a considerable bureaucratic burden on pathology departments.

The direct £5.8 million costs of the Authority are much less than the indirect costs of pathology personnel and the time they must put aside to comply. Public opinion might make it difficult to disband this Authority now, but it is worthy of consideration. Is it value for money, do patients benefit in any way, and would their safety be compromised if it was disbanded? These are questions that deserve close examination.

Similarly, there are several bodies that could be merged or simply taken into NHS England. Could, for example, the Health Services Safety Investigations, NHS Counter Fraud Authority Body, and the National Data Guardian be merged? In any case, each of these bodies relies on other non-government bodies for information.

The DHSC is profligate in its recourse to external advisory bodies. They are very expensive, and much more thought should be given to whether the advice gained provides value for money. Governments have access to expert and 'free' advice from their select committees.

There are savings to be made to the exchequer that are dependent on increased investment in the NHS. Ensuring that people can return to productive work and pay taxes can follow improvements in their care. Obvious examples are reductions in waiting lists for hospital care and more rapid appointments for treatment in primary care. The example of the successful treatment of common mental illnesses – particularly anxiety and depression – has been the subject of thorough economic evaluation. Richard Layard has clearly demonstrated the financial gain made by the use of 'Talking Therapies'.[85, 121] A six-week course of cognitive behaviour therapy (CBT) ensures that about 50% of patients are able to return to full-time employment and a further 20% are improved. A course costs about £1,000 but the returns made from taxable work are some 25 times greater. However, only some 13% of eligible patients receive this care, and it is only through increased investment in psychologists that the returns will be made. Improving health by investing in health care not only benefits patients, it improves the country's finances.

Funding the Gap

Despite the success of a previous Chief Executive of the NHS, Simon Stevens, in leveraging extra funds for the NHS, the services remain seriously underfunded.

Whatever savings can be made by the pruning of existing bodies, it is inevitable that the need for more funding to meet the shortfall in NHS expenditure will have to be met by taxation of some sort.

Where this additional taxation will come from, at a time when it is anathema to both main political parties, has been impossible to discern.

A Hypothecated Tax

One method that deserves to be re-examined is a tax specifically hypothecated for health and social care. This depends on the untested presumption that the public would be supportive of a modest increase in tax if it was to be used specifically for health care. It is not an impossibility, however. Currently, National Insurance contributions disappear into the Treasury coffers but are used to pay for such needs as pensions and social security benefit schemes. If these insurance payments were diverted to fund health care alone, other taxes would inevitably have to rise. Nevertheless, this would fulfil what many of the population believe – that NI payments should be used primarily for health insurance – and they might be willing to offer an increased subscription.

Calculations suggest, however, that NI contributions, even if enhanced, would be insufficient to cover the costs of the services. It could be further increased if, for instance, everyone, regardless of age, made contributions. Pensioners who continue to earn an income would be required to contribute at the same rate as those below retirement age. This would have the additional benefit of sharing the cost of care by those who use the services most with the young who use it least.

I owe the idea of a hypothecated tax to my colleagues Lords Layard and Macpherson, but I present it here as one possible way forward.

I have no doubt that more funds will be required, but until the money is found, there is much that can and should be done to improve care, as I have described. We should not wait for the magic money tree to bear fruit. I hope the proposals I have made will go a little way towards meeting that end.

Summary of Proposals

There is a commonly expressed opinion that the NHS is a bottomless pit and that there will never be enough money available to run it. But money really does talk, and it spoke loudly when Tony Blair increased funding to match the rest of Europe, with remarkable results. Waiting lists disappeared, GP appointments improved, and patient satisfaction levels rose. But now it is clear that the services are again underfunded for what is required of them.

It is regarded as unrealistic now, with poor national productivity and a failing economy, to expect a major relief for the NHS. But there are ways in which money may be saved. For example, by pruning the many agencies working under the banner of the Department of Health and Social Care. There are welcome suggestions to cut the very high legal costs of litigation by the introduction of a no-fault compensation system. And it might be worth examining the roles of other bodies, such as the Human Tissue Authority. But more money will still be needed and a hypothecated tax for health is worthy of further examination.

There is also the need for a recognition in the Treasury that investment in a healthy workforce brings much-needed tax revenues. Nowhere is that more obvious than in the successful treatment of the very common conditions of anxiety and depression. These illnesses are a huge drain on benefit payments, but can be converted into tax gains from productive work by a modest investment in the relevant psychological therapists.

CHAPTER 12
CONCLUSION

In this book, I have suggested a number of ways in which the NHS and care in the community may be improved by focussing on the patients and those who care for them. I have avoided suggesting that a huge increase in funding is necessary or that a reorganisation of the management of the services is at all desirable. The founding principle of the NHS of 'free at the point of service', is widely admired and supported but now there are serious concerns that it is failing to provide an acceptable level of service. Failures are perceived as waiting lists for hospital care increase, limited access to primary care, and social and community care struggling to cope with demand.

Social and Community Care

Attention at the outset is required to social and community care where prevention and support can provide huge dividends for patients and society. The whole edifice of the NHS is dependent on the way we care for people in the community, yet these services are barely coping.

Three types of problem should be faced.

The burdensome bureaucracy faced by applicants for care leaves many frustrated and in despair. The complicated assessment processes should now be rationalised, simplified, and the current delays removed.

For those caring for their elderly or disabled family or friends at home, the current financial support is grossly inadequate and only available after applicants have been through a tedious and difficult application process. This resource, that is largely free to the country, provides enormous cost savings to the exchequer and should now be re-examined. Application processes should be rationalised and a fair rate of compensation given.

Most importantly, attention must now be paid to the conditions of service that care workers in care homes suffer under. Poor pay is only one problem that should be corrected now. A lack of a registered professional qualification after an approved training programme should now be corrected. I describe ways in which that, and the necessary career progression, can be achieved. Only in this way will the large number of staff vacancies and the high rate of staff loss be corrected.

Revisiting the Dilnot proposals to reduce the burden on applicants for care should be considered, but priority should be given to improving the retention of care workers, health visitors, and district nurses, all of whom are sadly depleted.

Consideration should also be given to introducing a 'National Care Commission'.

Primary Care

Long delays for appointments to see a GP are far too common. The number requesting appointments has increased as the number of GPs has fallen. GPs are retiring early under the strain.

To improve primary care, the non-clinical load of bureaucracy that is taking up far too much time must be reduced. Improved support services should be provided in each practice to reduce this load. IT systems work well in many practices but high quality IT should be spread more widely and should increasingly be made to link with hospital and community services. Patients should be given direct and automatic access to their results and records. Too often they are denied this.

The further development of Community Diagnostic Centres for groups of GPs in larger conurbations is a valuable development but more attention should be given to the continuity of care that is threatened by this development.

The role of AI in primary care has potential but will require careful evaluation.

There is a desperate need to enhance the retention of GPs and to increase the time they can spend in direct clinical care. I discuss how this might be achieved.

Secondary, Hospital Care

Many problems arising in hospital care, including long waiting lists, delayed discharges, and cancelled operations, are due to defects in primary, and community and social care, yet these services are managed and funded separately. While this continues, their problems must be dealt with separately, too.

Patient care is best provided where the caring professions work as teams. This is no longer the norm and it is vital that efforts should be made to re-introduce teamworking. Ward rounds, at which doctors, trainees, and senior nurses all attend should be re-introduced on a regular basis. Formalised ward rounds and regular staff meetings should be brought back and will be dependent on more effective clinical leadership.

Attention should be given by Medical Royal Colleges and Postgraduate Deans to the question of whether current disruptive training programmes are achieving their aims.

Nursing career structures should be re-examined and the nursing sister in charge of a ward should be given greater authority, a more permanent career leadership role, and an appropriate pay reward.

Nursing Associate and Auxiliary posts should be given greater prominence in recruitment drives to fill the gap in non-university educated trainees.

Repairs to the hospital physical estate are urgently needed, but it is the staff difficulties that require even more effort. Greater appreciation of staff, for example by providing food catering out of hours, and by attention to car parking charges, could help improve the recruitment and retention of critical staff.

Mental Health Services

Parity of esteem between mental and physical health services is far from being achieved.

Anxiety and depression are extremely common, yet patients wait too long to receive the valuable services that are available. Talking therapies are very effective and at least 50% of patients are able to return to productive work after six weeks of therapy. Greater investment in clinical psychologists would yield valuable dividends to the treasury. Similarly, attention should now be given to enhancing the care and treatment of patients with drug addiction and anti-social behaviour. This is an aspect of care that is sorely underresourced.

Too many patients with autism and ADHD are locked away in mental hospitals. In advance of an awaited Mental Health Act, they should now be released to their families or care in the community.

Mental Health nursing is not regarded as an attractive occupation. This should now be corrected by improving conditions of service, prospects for career progression, and relevant pay awards to increase recruitment and retention.

The mental health of children is a key determinant of health in later life. Greater effort to detect and manage mental disturbances in childhood will require the greater involvement of teachers in this endeavour.

Maternity Services

CQC assessments of maternity care reveal a picture of variable and too often poor standards of care. There is evidence, too, of worse outcomes amongst black and other ethnic minority mothers. Many of the problems can be ascribed to poor levels of staffing and low morale. Solutions depend on making midwifery a more satisfying career. Attention should now be paid to improving career prospects and clinical leadership roles, and to repairing the continuing divisions between midwives and obstetricians. Mutual distrust is unhelpful and the Nursing and Midwifery Council and the Royal College of Obstetricians should re-examine how divisions can be repaired.

The health of neonates clearly influences health in later life. They should be given the best start in life and attention must be given to correcting the discrepancies in survival of babies (and mothers) from black and ethnic minority backgrounds.

Public Health

Few people are unaware that smoking, drinking too much alcohol, and eating high calorie foods can damage their health. So, more advice on healthy living is of limited value.

Government action has had a positive effect on smoking and it will require more such action to influence unhealthy behaviour. Pressure on industry to reduce the sugar content of soft drinks and the salt and sugar content of other foods is necessary. Limiting the advertising of fast foods and of outlets near to schools should be brought forward. Alcohol consumption falls as duty rises. The incidence of severe liver disease falls in the years after a rise in duty and governments should control their reluctance to raise duty in line with inflation.

The response to the Covid outbreak was clearly sub-optimal. Efforts should be made to re-instate the network of public health laboratories across the country to monitor food and water supplies and to track and trace outbreaks of infectious diseases. The lack of such facilities exposed us to the poor response to Covid.

Greater and more sophisticated efforts should be made to counter the negative propaganda levelled against vaccination and immunisation. The use of modern electronic techniques to target vulnerable populations would be valuable.

Health visitors are in the front line in drawing attention to hazards in the community that can lead to poor health, including poor housing and unsanitary conditions. There are dangers in allowing the falling numbers of health visitors to continue and steps should be taken to reverse this damaging drop.

Trust and Mistrust

Patients rely on the trust that they place in their carers, but trust is increasingly threatened. Regaining trust once it has been lost is extraordinarily difficult, yet mistrust is widely felt. Mistrust between government and the caring professions can only be assuaged with more inspired leadership on both sides. It will take time. Mistrust between doctors and nurses comes from a loss of the team spirit and poor communication. Efforts described earlier to improve teamworking will be necessary.

Improving trust at several levels is vital for patient care and it requires specific effort at the local level to stimulate it.

Medical Research

The UK has much to be proud of in its successes in medical research. But it could do much better if it could overcome the barriers to progress.

Clinical research is hampered by the pressures on clinicians to provide patient care at the expense of research time. Suggestions to lighten the clinical load and provide time for research are interesting but are unlikely to be achieved without a substantial increase in the number of clinicians, both trainees and established staff.

Some relief for researchers could come from reducing the bureaucratic hurdles that have to be overcome in gaining permission for research. Encouragement for GPs to allow the use of data derived from their patients for research is vital for much clinical research. Government inducements and reassurances about the safety and confidentiality of the use of patient data will be necessary.

Attention should be paid by the GMC to a more flexible approach to encourage senior overseas clinical researchers to come to work in the UK.

Reorganisation of the NHS

It may be asked whether any of the frequent efforts to reorganise the structure of the NHS have been responsible for any improvements in the care of patients.

I have not put forward any suggestion that we should undertake a further reorganisation.

The only structural change worth promotion is one that sees the full integration of the NHS, primary care, and social and community care. The new Integrated Care Boards are a potentially useful first step, but the best way in which integration can be made to occur is at the local level by those working at the coal face. High quality leadership at the hospital trust and local authority level is where it should begin. It has been shown to be effective in a small number of sites. It now needs strong government support for it to be fully achieved.

Funding Matters

That more funding is required is undeniable and there is little evidence to support the contention that the health service is a bottomless pit. Money does talk and spoke loudly when Tony Blair's Government increased funding to match the EU average percentage spend.

Sadly, poor national productivity and a failing economy now leaves little hope of a major government funding initiative. There are ways, however, in which savings may be made.

Pruning the many agencies and other bodies working under the banner of the Department of Health and Social Care would be a useful start. There are just too many of them. There are welcome suggestions that the high legal costs of litigation can be reduced by the introduction of no-fault compensation. This should be encouraged. A closer assessment of the benefits and direct and indirect costs of such other bodies as the Human Tissue Authority is worthwhile.

But more money will still be needed and the suggestion of a hypothecated tax, perhaps based on an extended National Insurance scheme devoted solely to health care is worthy of close examination.

Governments should know that a healthy workforce is a productive one. They should recognise that investment in health care will get people back to work quicker and revenues would rise. It is particularly the case that improving care in the community and in mental health have a demonstrable impact on reducing the numbers of unemployed.

Many proposals in this book do not require more funding but some do, and the Government should think of the dividends it could gain.

FURTHER READING

Britnell, M., *In Search of the Perfect System,* Palgrave, London, 2016.

Chandler, D., *Free and Equal. What Would a Fair Society Look Like?* Allen Lane, London, 2023.

Dalley, G., *Caring in Crisis: The Search for Reasons and Post-Epidemic Remedies*, Palgrave Macmillan, London, 2022.

Exworthy, M., Mannion, R., & Powel, M., *The NHS at 75: The State of UK Health Policy*, Policy Press, London, 2023.

Hardman, I., *Fighting for Life*, Penguin, London, 2023.

Kenway, E., *Who Cares: The Hidden Crisis of Caregiving and How to Solve It,* Headline, London, 2023.

Layard, R., & Clark, D. M., *Thrive: The Power of Evidence-based Psychological Therapies*, Allen Lane, London, 2014.

Layard, R., *Happiness: Lessons From a New Science*, Allen Lane, London, 2005.

Lister, J., & Davis, J., *NHS Under Siege: The Fight to Save It In The Age of Covid*, Merlin Press, London, 2011.

Marmot, M., *Status Syndrome: How your Place on the Social Gradient Directly Affects Your Health*, Bloomsbury, London, 2004.

Marmot, M., *The Health Gap: The Challenge of an Unequal World*, Bloomsbury, London, 2015.

McCartney, M., *The Patient Paradox: Why Sexed Up Medicine is Bad for You*, Pinter and Martin, London, 2012.

Paton, C., *NHS Reform and Health Politics in the UK*, Palgrave Macmillan, London, 2022.

Seaton, A., *Our NHS: A History of Britain's Best Loved Institution*, Yale University Press, New Haven and London, 2023.

Thomas, C., *The Five Health Frontiers: A New Radical Blueprint*, Pluto Press, London, 2022.

Timmins, N., *Glaziers & Window Breakers: The Role of the Secretary of State for Health in Their Own Words*, Health Foundation, London, 2015.

Warner, N., *A Suitable Case for Treatment*, Grosvenor House, London, 2011.

Whittaker, P., *What is a Doctor?* Canongate, London, 2023.

Yuille, M., & Ollier, B., *Saving Sick Britain: Why we need the 'Health Service'*, Manchester University Press, Manchester, 2021.

ENDNOTES

[1] A Report Into The State of Health and Social Care in Britain Today, *The Times Health Commission*, February 2024.

[2] Rise of the Month-Long Wait Just to See Your GP, *The Times*, 16 December 2023.

[3] Adapting The NHS to the Needs of a New Era: At 75, Britain's Feted Health Service is Struggling to Cope With Demand, *Financial Times*, 4 July 2023.

[4] A&E Delays Put Patients in Danger, Says Leading Doctor, *The Times*, 5 September 2023.

[5] Britnall, M., *In Search of the Perfect System*, Palgrave MacMillan, London, 2016.

[6] Marr, A., *The New Statesman*, 26 May 2023.

[7] Trends in Patient-to-Staff Numbers at GP Practices in England: 2022, *Office of National Statistics*, 9 December 2022.

[8] A&E Attendances and Emergency Admissions 2022-23, *NHS England*, March 2023.

[9] British Social Attitudes, NHS and Social Care, *National Centre for Social Research*, 2022.

[10] Morris, J., Schlepper, L., Dayan, M., Jeffries, D., Maguire, D., & Merry, L., Public Satisfaction with The NHS and Social Care in 2022, *King's Fund Report*, 29 March 2023.

[11] National Life Table – Life Expectancy in the UK, *Office for National Statistics*, 2020-2022.

[12] Raleigh, V., What is Happening to Life Expectancy in England? *King's Fund Report*, 9 August 2022.

[13] House of Lords Debate on The Future of Adult Social Care, *Hansard*, Column 358, 30 March 2023.

[14] A "Gloriously Ordinary Life"; Spotlight on Adult Social Care, *House of Lords, Adult Social Care Committee, Report of Session 2022-23*, 8 December 2022.

[15] An Ageing Society Cannot Turn its Back on Social Care Any Longer, *Financial Times*, 10 June 2023.

[16] The State of the Adult Social Care Sector and Workforce in England, Key Findings 2022/23, *Skills for Care*, October 2023.

[17] Mind Reveals True Extent of Crisis in Mental Healthcare with More than 17,000 Reports of Serious Incidents in Past Year Alone, *Mind*, 10 October 2023, https://www.mind.org.uk/news-campaigns/news/mind-reveals-true-extent-of-crisis-in-mental-healthcare-with-more-than-17-000-reports-of-serious-incidents-in-past-year-alone/

[18] Your Choices in the NHS, *NHS*, 10 May 2023.

[19] One in Eight Britons Pay for Private Health Services, Survey Shows, *The Guardian*, 17 April 2023.

[20] Anandaciva, S., How Does the NHS Compare to The Health Care Systems of Other Countries? *King's Fund Report*, 26 June 2023.

[21] Rebolledo, I., & Charlesworth, A., How Does UK Health Spending Compare Across Europe Over the Last Decade? *The Health Foundation Report*, 16 November 2022.

[22] Health Services in Western Europe, *Office of Health Economics*, London, 1963.

[23] Europe Struggles to Revive Health Services after Pandemic, *Financial Times*, 10 May 2023.

[24] Israel Facing Acute Shortage of Physicians, *Jerusalem Post*, 2 June 2023.

[25] The State of Health Care and Adult Social Care in England 2022/23, *CQC Report*, 20 October 2023,

www.cqc.org.uk/publications/major-report/state-care/2022-2023

[26] Public Expenditure Statistical Analysis, *HM Treasury*, 2022.

[27] Boccarini, G., Stevenson, G., Sameen, H., & Shebavnekar, N., Adult Social Care Funding Pressures: Estimated Costs to Meet Growing Demand and Improve Services in England, *The Health Foundation*, 25 September 2023.

[28] Myers, R., District Nursing – It's Not Just an Injection, *King's Fund Blog*, 13 September 2016.

[29] McKellar, L., *Report: Association of Directors of Adult Social Services, Spring Survey 2021*.

[30] Ombudsman Stats Show Stark Reality of Life in England in 2023, *Local Government and Social Care Ombudsman*, July 2023.

[31] Reeves, C., Islam, A., & Gentry, T., The State of Health and Care of Older People in England 2023, *Age UK*, July 2023.

[32] Inequalities in Age and Standardised Mortality Rates, *The Health Foundation*, 6 January 2022.

[33] The New Statesman, Pg 24, 1 September 2023.

[34] Local Dementia Statistics, *Alzheimer's Society*, 2022.

[35] Carers Allowance, Benefits 2023-24, *Age UK*, 5 October 2023.

[36] Social Care: The Time Bomb No Political Party Wants to Touch, *The Times*, 28 July 2023.

[37] Rolewicz, L., Palmer, B., & Lobont, C., The NHS Workforce in Numbers, *Nuffield Trust*, 7 February 2023.

[38] Hunter, W., Health Visitor Shortages Leaving Primary Care 'Overwhelmed', *Nursing in Practice*, 7 June 2023.

[39] ADASS Spring Survey 2023, Final Report, *Adult Social Services*, 21 June 2023.

[40] Abrahams, C., Age UK Comment in Response to The Care Quality Commission (CQC) Annual Assessment of the State of Health and Adult Social Care in England Looking at the Quality of Care Over the Past Year, *Age UK*, 20 October 2023.

[41] Dilnot, A., Fairer Care Funding, *The Report of the Commission on Funding of Care and Support*, July 2011.

[42] Sutherland, S., With Respect to Old Age: Long Term Care – Rights and Responsibilities, *Royal Commission on Long Term Care*, The Stationery Office, 1999.

[43] People at The Heart of Care, Adult Social Care White Paper, *Department of Health and Social Care*, December 2021.

[44] Next Steps to Put People at The Heart of Care, *Department of Health and Social Care*, 4 April 2023.

[45] Reforming Adult Social Care in England, *National Audit Office*, 10 November 2023.

[46] Care Home Bed Availability, *Nuffield Trust*, 27 April 2023.

[47] Learner, S., Care Home Trends: 2022 Saw Numbers of UK Care Homes Decline, *Care Homes UK*, 19 September 2023.

[48] Social Care 360: Providers, Care Home Places, *King's Fund*, 1 March 2023.

[49] Karim, H., Care Home Costs and Care Fees on Average, *Lottie*, February 2024.

[50] Berg, V., Care Home Fees and Costs: How Much Do You Pay? *Care Home*, 22 January 2024, https://www.carehome.co.uk/advice/care-home-fees-and-costs-how-much-do-you-pay

[51] Workforce Intelligence, *Skills for Care*, https://www.skillsforcare.org.uk/Adult-Social-Care-Workforce-Data/Workforce-intelligence/Home.aspx

[52] Overseas Staff 'Exploited and Trapped' at UK Care Home, *BBC News*, 18 December 2023, https://www.bbc.co.uk/news/uk-67684417

[53] State of Care 2022/23, The State of Health Care and Adult Social Care in England, *Care Quality Commission*, October 2023.

[54] Whitaker, P., *What is a Doctor?* Canongate, London, 2023.

[55] Young, H., Unsustainable Workload, Part-time Working and Portfolio Careers: Results of the GP Trainee Survey, *King's Fund*, 9 October 2023.

[56] Pressures in General Practice Data Analysis, *British Medical Association*, 16 February 2024.

[57] The Future of General Practice, House of Commons Health and Social Care Committee, *Fourth Report of Session 2022-23*, 20 October 2022.

[58] Brennan, N., Langdon, N., Bryce, M., Gale, T., Knapton, A., Burns, L., & Humphries, N., Drivers of International Migration of Doctors to and from the United Kingdom, *Final Report for General Medical Council*, ITT GMC996, July 2021.

[59] Ferreira, T., Collins, A. M., Feng, O., Samworth, R. J., & Horvath, R., Career Intentions of Medical Students in the UK: a National Cross-sectional Study (AIMS Study), *BMJ Open*, 13, Article 9, 2023, https://doi.org/10.1136/bmjopen-2023-075598

[60] Evidence Standards Framework for Digital Health Technologies, *NICE*, 9 August 2022.

[61] NHS Medical Staffing Data Analysis, *British Medical Association*, 25 January 2024.

[62] The GP Shortfall in Numbers, *The Health Foundation*, 30 June 2022.

[63] RCGP Responds to Labour's Latest Report on GP Practice Closures, *RCGP*, 11 July 2023.

[64] Why Are So Many GPs Shutting Up Shop? *The Guardian*, 27 September 2023.

[65] Rolewicz, L., Chart of the Week: Which Areas of England Have The Highest Number of Patients per GP? *Nuffield Trust*, 29 October 2021.

[66] Darzi, A., *High Quality Care for All. NHS Next Stage Review, Final Report*, The Stationery Office, 30 June 2008.

[67] Baker, C., NHS Key Statistics for England, *House of Commons Library*, 15 November 2023.

[68] Managing NHS Backlogs and Waiting Times in England, *House of Commons Committee on Public Accounts, 38th Report of Session 2022-23*, 2 February 2023.

[69] The Crisis in the NHS is Largely a Crisis in Older People's Preventive Care, and If We Are to Avoid Another Catastrophic Winter in Nine Months' Time, We Need to Act Now to Fix It Warns Age UK, *Age UK*, 17 February 2023.

[70] A&E Waiting Times, *QualityWatch*, Nuffield Trust, 15 February 2024.

[71] Data Show 1.65 Million Patients in England Faced 12-hour Waits from Time of Arrival in A&Es in 2022, *Royal College of Emergency Medicine*, 28 February 2022.

[72] Jones, S., Moulton, C., Swift, S., Molyneux, P., Black, S., Mason, N., Oakley, R., & Mann, C., Association Between Delays to Patient Admission from the Emergency

Department and All-cause 30-day Mortality, *Emergency Medicine Journal*, 39, 2022.

[73] Layard, R., *Happiness: Lessons from a New Science*, Allen Lane, London, 2005.

[74] NHS Staff Survey 2022, *National Results Briefing*, March 2023.

[75] Chandler, D., *Free and Equal*, Allen Lane, London, 2023.

[76] Dewar, H. A., The Hospital Nurse After Salmon and Briggs, *Journal of the Royal Society of Medicine*, 71, 399-405, June 1978.

[77] Palmer, W., Rolewicz, L., & Dobsworth, E., Waste Not, Want Not: Strategies to Improve the Supply of Clinical Staff to the NHS, *Nuffield Trust*, September 2023.

[78] Farrah, M., Does a Fall in Degree Applicants Signal the End for the Current Nursing Staffing Model? *Nurses.co.uk*, 12 September 2023.

[79] Over 50 New Surgical Hubs Set to Open Across England to Help Burst the Covid 19 Backlog, *UK Government Press Release*, 26 August 2022.

[80] The Case for Surgical Hubs, *Royal College of Surgeons, Strategy Unit*, 2023.

[81] Grey, P., Nurses are Highly Skilled Workers and Should be Paid as Such, *New Statesman, Spotlight*, 13 October 2023.

[82] Aiken, L. H., Sloane, D. M., Bruyneel, L., Van den Heede, K., Griffiths, P., Busse, R., *et al.* Nurse Staffing and Education and Hospital Mortality in Nine European Countries: a Retrospective Observational Study, *Lancet*, 383. (9931)1824-1830, 26 February 2014.

[83] Baker, C., & Kirk-Wade, E., Mental Health Statistics: Prevalence, Services and Funding in England, *House of Commons Library*, 13 March 2023.

[84] Layard, R., & Clark, D. M., *Thrive*, Allen Lane, London, 2014.

[85] Layard, R., *Hansard*, Column 1754, 8 February 2024.

[86] Welfare Spending: Disability Benefits, *Office for Budget Responsibility*, November 2023.

[87] Welfare Trends Report, *Office for Budget Responsibility*, January 2019.

[88] *Anorexia Nervosa – Highest Mortality Rate of Any Mental Disorder: Why?* Accessed December 2023, www.eatingdisorderhope.com/information/anorexia

[89] Crisis Care Services 'Under-resourced, Understaffed and Overstretched' Mind Looks at Damning Crisis Care Statistics, *Mind*, Accessed 29 December 2023, www.mind.org.uk/news

[90] Concerning Pressures on NHS Mental Health Staff Causing Vicious Cycle of Staff Shortages, *UK Parliament Public Accounts Committee*, 21 July 2023.

[91] Number of Autistic People in Mental Hospitals: Latest Data, *National Autistic Society*, 17 February 2022.

[92] Bannister, R., Underfunded Mental Healthcare in the NHS: the Cycle of Preventable Distress Continues, *British Medical Journal*, 375, 2706, 2021.

[93] Bell, A., & Pollard, A., No Wrong Door: A Vision for Mental Health, Autism and Learning Disability Services in 2032, *NHS Confederation*, 2 December 2022.

[94] Stanton, E., The Case for Change in British Mental Healthcare, *Journal of the Royal Society of Medicine*, 107(4) 135, 2014.

[95] National Survey Shows Some Improvement in Maternity Experiences, But Help Not Always Available When Needed, *Care Quality Commission*, 9 February 2024.

[96] Safe Staffing: The Impact of Staffing Shortages in Maternity and Neonatal Care, *All-Party Parliamentary Group on Baby Loss*, 21 October 2022.

[97] Mothers and Babies: Reducing Risk through Audit and Confidential Enquiries (MBRRACE-UK). *Saving Lives, Improving Mothers' Care State of the Nation Surveillance, State of Care Report*, 20 October 2023.

[98] *Hansard*, Column 854, 25th January 2024.

[99] Debt, Dole, Worry: Midwives Facing Triple Whammy Threat, *Royal College of Midwives Report*, 7 October 2020.

[100] 17 New NHS Centres Dedicated to Preventing Maternity Deaths and Complications, *NHS Announcement*, 19 March 2023.

[101] Kimm, S. Y. S., Fetal Origins of Adult Disease: the Barker Hypothesis Revisited-2004, *Current Opinion in Endocrinology & Diabetes*, 11(4):192-196, August 2004.

[102] Marmot, M., *The Health Gap*, Bloomsbury, London, 2015.

[103] Independent Inquiry into Inequalities in Health, *The Acheson Report*, The Stationery Office, 26 November 1998.

[104] Government Preparedness for the Covid 19 Epidemic: Lessons for Government Risk, *House of Commons Committee of Public Accounts, 46th Report of Session 2021-22*, 23 March 2022.

[105] The Public Health Response by UK Governments to Covid 19, *British Medical Association*, 2 October 2023.

[106] Pini, P., PHLS celebrates Golden Jubilee, *The Lancet*, 338, 9038, 16 November 1996.

[107] Buck, D., & Ewbank, L., What is Social Prescribing? *The King's Fund*, 4 November 2020.

[108] Hawkes, N., More Than 30 Health Quangos May Be Axed by UK Coalition Government, *British Medical Journal*, 24 September 2010.

[109] Khaton, T., Littlejohn, P., & Hunter, D. J., "Bonfire of the Qangos" – Let's Make a Pyre of this Perennial Ritual, *NIHR*, 24 May 2022.

[110] Commercial Clinical Trials in the UK: The Lord O'Shaughnessy Review, *Gov.UK*, 26 May 2023.

[111] Future-Proofing UK Health Research: A People-Centred, Co-ordinated Approach, *The Academy of Medical Sciences Report*, January 2020.

[112] Timmins, N., *Glaziers and Window Breakers: The Role of the Secretary of State for Health in their Own Words*, Health Foundation, 2015.

[113] Judt, T., *Ill Fares the Land*, Penguin, London, 2010.

[114] Commissioning, *House of Commons Health Committee, Fourth Report*, 18 March 2010.

[115] Commissioning, *House of Commons Health Committee, Third Report*, 13 January 2011.

[116] Paton, C., *NHS Reform and Health Politics in the UK*, Palgrave Macmillan, London, 2022.

[117] Timmins, N., *The Most Expensive Breakfast in History: Revisiting the Wanless Review 20 Years On*, Health Foundation, London, 2021.

[118] Warner, N., *A Suitable Case for Treatment*, Grosvenor House, London, 2011.

[119] Gov.UK Departments, Agencies and Public Bodies, www.gov.uk/government/organisations

[120] NHS Litigation Reform, *House of Commons, Health and Social Care Committee Enquiry*, 28 April 2022.

[121] Baker, C., & Kirk-Wade, E., Mental Health Statistics: prevalence, services and funding in England, *House of Commons Library*, 13 March 2023.

Other Books from the Publisher

The Secret Magistrate

Every criminal case starts in a magistrates' court, and most end there. Last year, the 14,000 magistrates of England & Wales dealt with almost 1.4 million cases.

But, what exactly does a magistrate do, who are they, and how are they recruited and trained? Are they out-of-touch and unrepresentative, or still fit for purpose with a role to play in today's increasingly sophisticated and complex judicial system?

The Secret Magistrate takes the reader on an eye-opening, behind-the-scenes tour of a year in the life of an inner-city magistrate. Chapters cover a variety of cases including the disqualified driver who drove away from court, the Sunbed Pervert, and Fifi the Attack Chihuahua.

Master Your Chronic Pain: A Practical Guide

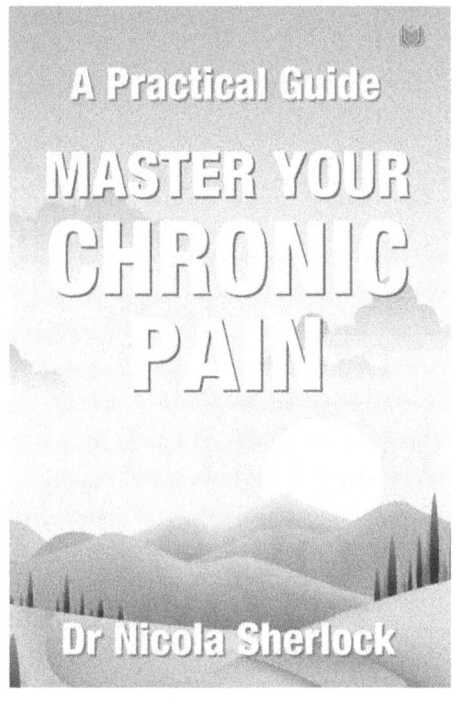

Chronic pain is a huge problem. It is estimated that between one third and one half of the adult population in the UK live with pain. In turn, many people struggle to manage their pain; they report that it affects nearly every aspect of their lives, and that they feel held captive by it.

Furthermore, the emotional impact of pain has been increasingly recognised, and it is recommended that treatments for chronic pain no longer rely on medication alone. However, it is difficult to find relatable, easy-to-understand information on the non-medical aspects of pain management.

Master Your Chronic Pain adopts a holistic view of pain. Each chapter looks at a different aspect of pain management, from the benefits of mindfulness meditation to overcoming a fear of exercise to strategies for improving sleep. The emotional impact of pain is discussed, and practical tips for managing stress, worry, and low mood are given. Strategies for managing thoughts and emotions are explored, and the impact of pain on relationships is examined. This book uses principles from Acceptance and Commitment Therapy (ACT) which has been established as a highly effective therapeutic approach in the management of chronic pain.